Becoming a Butterfly

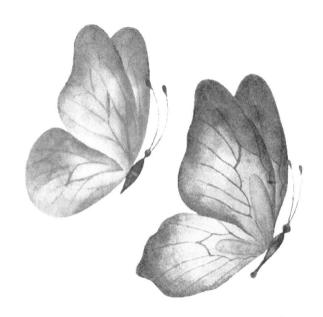

By
Kylie Beaudry & Kristy Haigh

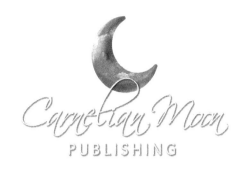

PUBLISHING

Published by Carnelian Moon Publishing, Inc. Ottawa, Ontario, Canada
Copyright © 2022 by Kylie Beaudry & Kristy Haigh, All rights reserved.

Special thanks to the Carnelian Moon Publishing Team: Editing by Magda Kacprzak , Cover Design by Tanja Prokop of Book Cover World, Interior Layout by The 2 Creative Minds Agency.

Edition 1, December, 2022,
eBook ISBN: 978-1-7387897-1-9
Paperback ISBN: 978-1-7387897-0-2

Table of Contents

Introduction

Dedicated to our 20-year-old selves
and to every person doing the work to become a beautiful and magical butterfly.

Introduction

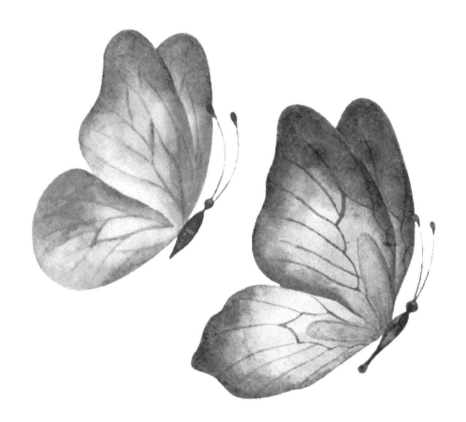

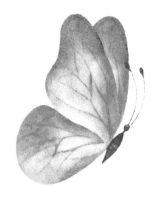

As we begin

with gratitude from Kristy

WHEN I GOT MY DIAGNOSIS of anxiety and minor depression, I felt like it was a death sentence. I watched movies about people who'd gotten their diagnosis and went on a complete downward spiral. My doctor said that he could get me on antidepressants right away.

I felt like someone had knocked all the air out of my lungs. My chest felt heavy and my heart was thumping hard against my rib cage. I thought it was going to tear my chest open and leave me lifeless in the doctor's office. I didn't want to take medication. It scared me, but I thought that if I didn't go with it, my life might be at stake. I felt torn between the urge to do what would be the logical solution and what was in my heart that was urging me to find another way.

With immense courage, I spoke up.

"I don't feel like medication is the right path for me, but I'm worried that my health will continue to decline if I don't do something."

"But, I'm worried that I'll destroy myself if I don't stop this." To this day I'm grateful for my courage to voice my doubts and for my doctor, who could understand my reservations about taking medication. My doctor offered me alternatives; he gave me contact information to see a counselor, and he suggested I try different activities and exercises. He also suggested watching my food and what I was consuming because certain foods could not only make you feel tired and bloated, but also affect your moods. After hearing this, I decided not to take the medication. It scared me that I needed it, but I knew deep down that it wasn't meant to be a part of my journey.

I had to keep myself accountable. I went through 3 counselors to find the one that worked for me. Or better yet, with me. My first counselor didn't allow me to talk about what I was experiencing, but gave me a list of medications that I SHOULD be on and lots of HOMEWORK that they printed off for me to do. I would leave each session with about 26 pages of activities and a medication list that was faxed to my doctor.

Even though I continued telling them I didn't think medication was meant for me, they would tell me I wouldn't get better without it.

After a month of sessions, I sought out another counselor. This time I had sessions and exercises which weren't that overwhelming. However, I stopped going to this counselor because they told me that there wasn't anything wrong with me and I was just seeking attention.

To someone with a mental health illness, this was disheartening. I felt as though my stomach was trying to escape my body.

Here I was at 21, fearing what people would assume when I told them I had a mental illness and hearing, "You just want attention," from a professional. My heart sank as I realized I wasn't being taken seriously. I hated myself. I felt like I'd wasted this person's time that could have been spent with someone who really needed their help. I had told no one about my diagnosis except my mom, my doctor, and then the counselor. After that session, I left and didn't go back. I spent the next six months hiding.

I did other things that my doctor had suggested. It led me to the practice of yoga, and even though I was training with a group of people, I felt in solitude with my mind.

What counted was the present moment, where I didn't have to do anything but wait for the next pose. I would leave my classes feeling empowered. I also joined a Pilates class, and started scheduling gym time. Later, I went back to my doctor and he asked how things were going.

Soft tears slid down my face as I commented I was better. He asked why I was crying and I just said that I felt anxious all the time except when I was at the gym. He also wanted to know how the counseling was going, and I told him I no longer went to see anyone.

He was curious to know why, so I evasively said it didn't work out , and that the last counselor had said there wasn't anything wrong with me, that I just wanted attention. My doctor seemed disappointed and suggested that I try speaking with my school counselor. He said that sometimes we need to keep looking until we find someone we're compatible with, similar to how you might choose your hairdresser.

I took his advice and went to see a counselor at my university. Although I feared wasting someone's time again, and I felt apprehensive about making an appointment, I was so glad I did it. This counselor listened to me, really listened to me! They gave me "homework" designed in such a way that it felt like small bite-sized pieces. When I said I was anxious about wasting their time as I'd felt during my last experience, they told me that mental health didn't look the same for everyone and I should never be made to feel like I was wasting someone's time. Our sessions went well, I was led to some great spiritual authors, and the entire experience jump-started my healing journey.

By doing everything that was needed to keep me mentally healthy, I was able to retrain my brain, gently programming myself to believe that my health was a priority, and to start moving forward in my life instead of staying stagnant.

My diagnosis had felt like darkness so absolute. When you first get the diagnosis that you have anxiety and depression, you start to define yourself as such. You begin to take on this identity of an anxious and depressed being. It consumes you. I couldn't see past that early in my journey.

Have you ever heard the expression "what you focus on grows"? Well, my anxiety was what I was focused on. I'd created a world that was led by anxiety, a life of isolation by my design, an internal prison of my own making.

It was how I was identifying myself, "I can't do this because I have anxiety," or "I am so stressed". This was my story most of the time until I realized it didn't have to be. I could create a life of love, full of beautiful and abundant moments. I could rewrite this story.

For crying out loud, I wasn't even the main character in this story. I was the one who sometimes made appearances when something remotely happy happened. Can you guess who was taking the lead? That's right, anxiety was the star of this show. How sad is that?

It was like being in a toxic relationship, but instead of being with another person, I was with myself. The anxiety made all the decisions, all the plans, and I was living in a world where I was barely surviving. When you think of your one precious life, do you just want to survive it? No! You want to freaking LIVE it! Enjoy it. Feel it. Yes, feel! Really feel what it means to be alive.

How does one go from a life as a busy, anxious, and depressed mind to one that is no longer focused and defined by it? Well, this is our (mine & Kylie's) journey back to truly living. Though our experiences vary, mental health is just as important as your physical health; and we are here to guide you through what has helped us redefine ourselves. My loves, YOU aren't your anxiety or your depression. Our hope for you is that you can find at least one thing in our book that you can embody and get back to being the main character of your life. To transform from the caterpillar into that beautiful, soulful, vibrant butterfly.

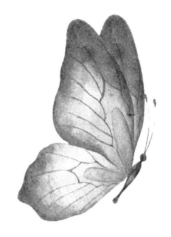

Coming together

in openness with Kylie

DEPRESSION AND ANXIETY are issues I struggle with. I don't want to say I'm depressed and anxious because I'm so much more than that. I'm a young woman. I'm compassionate.

I'm hardworking. I'm creative and I'm intelligent. I'm a terrible cook, and I'm a horrible singer. That's who I am. Depression and anxiety are a part of me, but they aren't all of me.

Although some days feel like all there is to me are my mental health struggles, there are many other days when I make it through the entire 24 hours, barely thinking about them. I'm on top of the world! The sun is shining! The butterflies are beautiful, there are rainbows... and there's a dark cloud... but that's in the distance. Right now, I'm soaring. Life is good.

Until I wake up the next day and can't get out of bed. That's why I call it a struggle. I have good days. And, I have bad days. But I always have days because I continue to push through, and I'm determined to live the fullest life possible regardless of the struggles I face.

Now, I'm sure you're wondering how the heck I do this. I'm by no means an expert on living with mental health issues, but I do consider myself an expert on persevering.

No matter the struggle or the way I feel, I make it through each day, and I'm here to tell you how I do this.

While Kristy has chosen the path of not taking medication, I went the other route.

I decided that I'd go through this journey by allowing pharmaceuticals to help me through it. That is not to say one way is better than the other, but you'll find a way that works for you. If you opt for pills and find you don't like them, you can always work with your doctor to come off them safely. However, if you decline treatment and decide later that you would like to try it, that's okay, too!

Have you ever been shopping and tried on a one size fits all dress? It might end up loose in the chest and too tight in the butt, and your head is poking out strangely like a turtle poking out of its shell. It looks great on the mannequin, but for some reason, you look like you belong on the What Not to Wear list. The mental health journey is like that. There's no one size fits all approach.

The journey on medication has been a wild ride for me. Like many people who take pills, it can take years before finding the right treatment for you. There may be side effects to adjust to. You may experience judgment from friends or family whom you confide in about the fact that you're taking pharmaceuticals. You may even feel self-judgment.

I remember thinking, "How messed up I am that I need something outside of myself to make me feel human!".

I spend my days hoping. I hope for world peace and for ending hunger. I hope for the elimination of poverty and for affordable homes. I hope for access to education for all. But with this book, I hope that you'll find some techniques that will assist you with persevering each day, no matter how hard the struggle may feel. Believe me, I understand how hard it can be hard. But, that's why we are sharing our journey with you.

But, you won't become a butterfly unless you're a caterpillar first.

"Depression and anxiety are a part of me, but they are not all of me."

Kylie

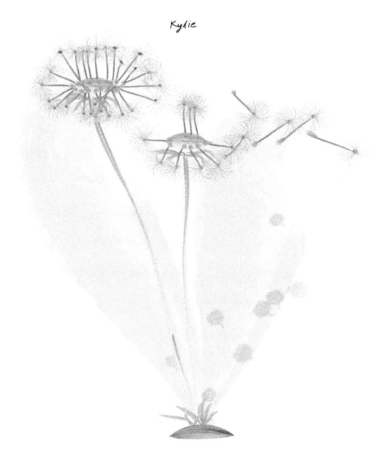

1

Nourishing Your Caterpillar

Written with love by Kylie

The basics, such as the key to any good outfit or the key to a productive and fulfilled life include — sleep, proper nutrition, and exercise — and are all fundamental in setting you up for success.

However, what are the essentials for becoming a butterfly? Let's dive in and find out!

Sleep

Sleep is important for your mental health. Without the right amount of sleep, it's harder to function, to get through the day, and to see things from a perspective that isn't tainted by your inner demons.

Professionals recommend between 7 and 9 hours of sleep per night. I'm no expert, but I have a pretty good feeling that most of us don't get this. We live in a world where sleep is viewed as wasteful, because we aren't working or producing anything. Nevertheless, I believe that a healthy amount of sleep is the most productive thing you can do for you.

Please, notice that I said, "a healthy amount". What would this healthy amount be exactly? Well, my dear, this is where you need to listen to your body. You should sleep if you are feeling exhausted! If you feel you haven't gotten enough rest, sleep! If you're feeling grouchy, sleep! Or eat something healthy to avoid those blood sugar imbalances that can lead to those "werewolf" moments of anger or annoyance.

If sleep is your chute, but you perceive yourself well rested and you get bored, get up! Go to get some fresh air and be active! Too much sleep isn't good for your mental health either. It'll take some trial and error, but you'll find the amount of sleep that works best for you.

It was recommended to me by a nutritionist that I try going to sleep and waking up at the same time each day between Monday and Friday. Provided that you work a weekday job, this habit could keep your body on a good schedule.

Let's assume that we currently go to bed and wake up at the same time each day, trying to get our 7-9 hours of sleep. However, how can we make sure that this time spent in bed is restful? This is where it gets fun, because this is all about what you like and it's about making yourself comfortable.

Let me paint you a picture. You're tucking yourself into your comfortable bed dressed in your favorite sheets and a pillow that has just the right amount of fluff. Your noise machine is on, ready to block out any disturbances. Your phone is in silent mode and out of sight; room temperature is perfect, too.

You take a few deep breaths to let go of the day you've had and then you close your eyes. How could you stop yourself from drifting off to sleep now? This sounds so peaceful!

Let's break it down!

We'll begin with your bed!

It needs to be comfy, and you'll want to have clean, soft sheets. Your pillow should also support your head perfectly. If you can't sleep without a blanket, have your favorite cozy blanket sprawled out on the bed.

Once your bed is made the way you like it, your room needs to be prepared for your sleep, too. First, close the curtains! A dark room will stimulate the production of melatonin, the naturally occurring chemical in your brain that helps you fall asleep quickly.

Also, make sure that the temperature is a touch on the cooler side. If you need a noise machine, get a noise machine! If you need a stuffed support animal, by all means hold one!

If you need a glass of water on your nightstand, make sure you have one ready for you!

One last note on your bed and bedroom! You've heard it before, your bedroom is for sleeping and sex only. Should you keep a TV here? Bad idea!

Let's talk about your phone now!

If you're trying to sleep and all you can hear is Buzz! Buzz!, your mind will not think about turning off. Instead, it is going to ponder over what messages there are on your phone that need to be responded to. Turn your phone off or put it on silent mode!

I recommend placing it in a drawer, leaving it in another room, or keeping it face down on your bedside table or somewhere close to the bed. It can be disturbing when you're in a dark room and the phone light flashes because you've received a notification. I highly suggest putting the phone in another part of the house, but I know a lot of us (me included) use our phones as an alarm clock, so I can understand keeping it in your room.

What activities are you doing before bed?

The experts I keep referring to recommend avoiding all types of screens before bed.

So, turn off those favourite reality show videos, stop scrolling through Instagram, and pick up a book instead! I like to read for a bit before going to sleep. It helps to slow my active mind and recover from the busy day I've had.

I would like to make one last point before moving on from sleep. I've recently gotten a puppy and I feel like some of you may be in the same situation. My puppy, Mocha, is adorable. She's a Chocolate Labrador Retriever, and she's full of love and life. I enjoy her sleeping in the bed with me. However, my body isn't a huge fan of Mocha snoozing right next to me. She moves around a lot; she licks herself, and now and then she barks, which isn't conducive to a good night's sleep.

Dog lovers come at me, but I put Mocha in a crate at nighttime so I can focus on my sleep. Call me self-centered, but it's okay to be selfish when it comes to our sleep.

Nutrition

I love chocolate. I enjoy chocolate cake, chocolate fudge, chocolate chip muffins, chocolate bars, and chocolate-covered strawberries (it's healthy because it's a fruit, right?).

If a meal or a dish has chocolate, sign me up! Chocolate goes great after a delicious carb-filled meal. Pasta? Love it. Pizza? Love it. Bread? Love it. Potatoes? Love it.

It's actually National Pizza Day as I'm writing this and you know what I'm having for dinner tonight, right? Pizza, get in my belly! You know I'm going to enjoy it!

Chocolate can even go on carbs. Have you ever had a dessert pizza? If you haven't, you must try it!

What do you call a chicken looking at a bowl of salad?
A chicken sees a salad!

Now, that I got that excitement out of the way, as much as these foods are delicious, they don't exactly have the nutritional value that you'd find in a Chicken Caesar salad. WAIT! Pause. Before you burn this book because you think I'm telling you that you should switch pizza or pasta for only salads and meats, just give me a minute to explain. If you still don't like what I'm saying, by all means, BURN BABY, BURN. But I have a feeling that you'll be on board.

Have you heard of the 80/20 rule? 80% of your diet should consist of healthy and nutritional meals. Do you know what the remaining 20% is? CHOCOLATE BABY!

This 80/20 plan sounds manageable. However, when life gets in full swing, the kids go to soccer practice or ballet you work late this week, and the cat needs to go to the vet. How the heck are you supposed to eat healthy? It takes time! It takes effort! You don't have time? I hear you. Trust me, I relate! I don't have that time, effort, energy, or willpower either. I don't even like cooking and now instead of throwing a pizza in the oven, I'm supposed to whip up a nice nutritional meal? Yeah, right!

How can I eat healthy while still living a busy life? My favorite word comes into play here. Preparation. That's right! You prepare in advance for the curve balls life throws at you.

Pick a day of the week that works for you, and cook a couple of meals you can throw in the freezer. Then, all you need to do throughout the week is exactly what you would do with your pizza. Take it out of the freezer and heat it up in the oven. A nutritious meal you don't have to cook in the evening because you've already done the preparation. It's a beautiful thing! I choose Sundays as my shopping and meal prep days, but you'll find a day that works for your schedule. It doesn't have to take the whole day either. Even a couple of hours can help set you up for success.

Perhaps I should have begun with this: there're many benefits to your mental health that proper nutrition can provide. When you're nourishing your body properly, you feel better and more energetic. This can be super helpful for supporting strong mental health. Junk food can make you feel lethargic and slow, which is the last thing you want to feel when struggling with depression.

Here's a list of foods I recommend for 80% of your diet. I'm not a nutritionist, but these have worked well for me.

- Eggs
- Meat
- Cheese
- Nuts

- Apples
- Bananas
- Yogurt
- Cottage cheese
- Protein shakes
- Dark chocolate
- Vegetables

As far as 20% of treats are concerned, I have a few suggestions for how to make them fit your lifestyle in a safe and healthy way.

- Eat out only once a week *(BONUS: this will help you save money, too!)*
- Watch the portion sizes of the snacks you have

In addition to mindful consideration of the nutrients you're fuelling your body with, remember too the importance of hydration. 70% of your body is made up of water, which is quite a lot. Many of the activities we do drain us of water, so it's important to replenish it regularly. Make sure you're actively drinking enough liquids throughout the day. This will also help you stay on track with healthy eating and you'll also feel better physically.

Nutrition is something I struggle with all day, every day, so I try not to be too hard on myself. We're all humans and we all have so much to learn. We gain new knowledge every day and we're doing the best we can. Remember that!

Exercise

I'm going to begin by letting you know right off the bat that I suck at this one. However, I have put measures in place to ensure that I'm as successful as I want to be because not liking something doesn't give you a free pass to avoid it. Sometimes things that are good for us are just what we need, and if it feels hard, that's probably because it is! That's life! Not everything is going to be easy, and accomplishing something that you had to work for will feel much more fulfilling.

I've designed the most elaborate workout schedules for myself. They are a work of art and frankly; I am appalled that I haven't been asked to put them in the Louvre yet.

They are color-coded and with stickers marking different types of workouts and schedules. Nevertheless, they always, always end up in the trash because I love making my workout schedules. I just suck at sticking to them.

That's why you need to find what works best for you. It took me MONTHS of getting up every day and trying before I learned what suited my needs. I persevered because exercise is important for mental health. It gives you something to focus on and put your energy into.

It works out your physical body and challenges your mind in a healthy way. If that isn't enough, it also gives you an excuse to eat treats sometimes and not to feel bad (which you shouldn't anyway, but I know we all do).

Do you want to know what works for me? Undoubtedly, our needs will differ, but joining a gym that has circuit-based classes turned out to be a perfect solution for me. I enjoy these classes because I feel like I'm challenging myself when I work out, and I appreciate their structured nature. I tried out a few gyms before I found a place where I felt comfortable. You need a spot where you feel like you belong, where you feel safe to challenge yourself, and where you're supported on your journey.

Physical exercise is a practice. You are meant to challenge yourself often, and push yourself to new levels. You are meant to try out things, fail, and then keep trying. You aren't meant to master.

Recap

essential guide posts

Sleep

- *7-9 hours/night*
- *No electronics*
- *Go to bed and wake up at the same time each day*

Nutrition

- *Watch portion sizes of the foods you eat*
- *Eat out no more than once a week*

Exercise

- *Daily, in a way that works for you*

Hygiene

- *Shower*

Let's personalize this! Make a list of your basic needs and then pin it some place where you'll see it every day. When you start feeling off, take a look at your list, and make sure you're meeting all your essential necessities.

Your Basic Needs List

List your 'non-negotiable' needs below

"Saying no can be therapeutic."

Kylie

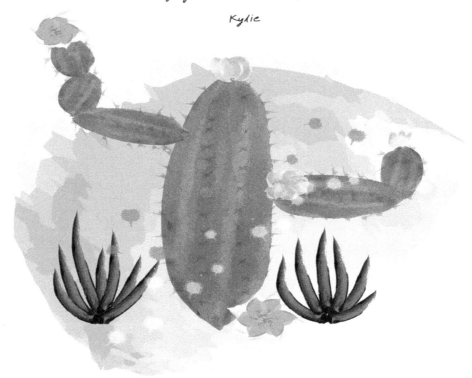

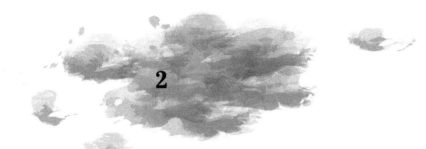

The Flutter of my Wings

Written with hope by Kylie

Imake handmade polymer clay earrings. I started this business in 2021 during the COVID-19 pandemic. When a lot of businesses were tragically forced to close, I was just getting started on this whirlwind experience.

As a business owner, it's important to branch out and take as many opportunities as possible. This is how you grow and how you meet people. This is how you expand so you can extend your community, increase sales, as well as increase your income.

Even opportunities that don't seem like something you would typically say yes to, you can accept, because they could lead to new experiences down the road. You might say yes to opportunities where you lose money with the hopes of making more money in the long run. You might say yes to opportunities last minute and then stay up the night before a market to prepare for it.

The point is, you're saying yes to opportunities because it's a door that is opening for you.

When I started Stella Jamieson Designs, I was searching for every door I could find.

I'd even knock on the doors that weren't open just to see if they would open for me. As a result, I ended up sending a message to the owner of Wild Heart Muskoka, a nifty little store in Port Sydney, Ontario, to find out if she would stock my earrings. We agreed to meet, and I drove over on my lunch break one day to check out the store and show her my earrings.

If you've never been to Muskoka, I highly recommend it! People come from all over the world to see what Muskoka has to offer – the landscape, the nature, the hiking trails, the water. It truly is a destination worth seeing. Whether you want to camp, glamp, cottage, or stay in a hotel, there are endless things to do and enjoy in Muskoka.

That being said, I lived about 15 minutes from Port Sydney at the time, and I'd never visited this small town next to mine. How sorry I felt! The road from the highway to Wild Heart Muskoka was beautiful, lined with trees on both sides, and a golf course constructed just next to it.

You drive over a bridge and past a park alongside the water's edge. The town itself is adorable, with a couple of restaurants and stores. You can call me the Grinch if you like, because my heart grew three sizes on that drive.

When I arrived at Wild Heart Muskoka, I show-cased my earrings, checked out the store, and I loved it! It was stocked with many gift ideas for all sorts of people. This wasn't just Wild Heart Muskoka saying yes to selling my earrings, but it was also me saying yes to allowing my earrings to be handled there, too. It was a mutual agreement.

About 3 weeks after I left my earrings in the store, I received a message from the owner asking me for more pieces because they were almost sold out! I jumped up and down with glee! To a small business owner, this was a dream come true. People were buying my earrings! People liked my earrings! People wanted more of my earrings! It was all because I had knocked on a door and when it opened for me, I took a look around... and I said YES!

Not long after I started selling my earrings at Wild Heart Muskoka, I decided to try out a new project for the summer: roller skating. Those of you who are athletic or well-balanced might not have much to think about this activity choice. For me, this was a big deal and I was determined to make it a thrilling adventure.

I tried skating on ice a bit when I was a child. Which Canadian kid hasn't? But roller skating? I'd never done that before, and I wasn't exactly known to be the most athletic of the bunch. I didn't care! Summer was four-month long in my eyes, and I had four months to learn how to get by on roller skates. No problem!

The first step to begin my training was buying the skates! Jibe Jewellery is a local store in Bracebridge, Ontario, which is located inside the Natural Food Market on the main street.

The owner, Christa, describes the store as a "boho general store." It's a gift shop with only the coolest gifts to choose from for your best pals. Christa hand makes the most beautiful jewellery that she offers there and she also sells roller skates.

When I noticed on social media that she was selling roller skates, I zipped over to Jibe in my speedy Impreza, and I immediately asked to try them on. I can't even recall if I said hello to her upon entrance. I was just so excited to check out new skates for this new hobby!

Shortly after, I was poorer by $200 but came waltzing out of Jibe with a big, pastel pink box that held the ticket to my summer hobby: my very first pair of roller skates!

I spent the entire afternoon skating up and down my hallway and watching videos online explaining how the heck these things worked. My purchase was a tad... shall we say impulsive?... but I had committed, and I was determined.

I posted a picture of my roller skates on my Stella Jamieson Designs Instagram page and tagged Jibe. Engaging in community connections? Check! When Christa realized I was the one who had bought the roller skates, and I was also a fellow artist, she reached out to see if I would be interested in roller skating with her and some of her friends.

What. A. Terrifying. Idea! I could barely go up and down my hallway in these skates, and now I was supposed to do it in public while trying to make a good impression on people! What had I gotten myself into?

There's only one way to get out of a hole when you've dug yourself into one, and that my friends, is to keep digging. That was exactly what I did. I told Christa I would love to meet up with her and her friends to roller skate some time. I convinced myself I would keep practicing every day to improve (oh, what a lie that was), and that this get-together could lead to further connections in the near future.

Soon after, Christa asked me if I would be interested in working at her shop one day per week. I debated this. I was working a full-time job already, and I was involved in many activities on the side; however, it was only five hours a week and extra money couldn't hurt. Besides, who knew where the opportunity would lead?

You have probably guessed it, but of course, I said I would help! Opening a new door? Check! I bet you think that's all there is to this story, but oh no, here is where it gets good.

On my first shift I was surprised by a lovely little welcome gift Christa had left for me with a handwritten note. She had also left a few tasks she was hoping I could do if I had time and she asked me if I might be interested in showcasing my earrings on one of the shelves in her shop. CUE INTERNAL SCREAMING.

I had said yes to trying a new hobby which led me to being offered a second job.

I had said yes to helping at Jibe which led Christa to asking me to showcase my earrings.

The more stores I could get my earrings into, the more people could see them and connect with me. This was business, connections with people, and I was doing it!

The more you say yes, the more you open yourself up to opportunities seeking you out. Let me repeat that. The more you say yes, the more you open yourself up to opportunities seeking you out!

Have you noticed how I said that opportunities were seeking you out? That's because I believe opportunities search for you, but you often close the door on them by saying no.

We look the other way or we say we are too busy, too tired, and too overworked. We make up reasons, some very legitimate, and we justify closing doors. But the point is, we close the door.

When you say yes, when you take that opportunity, it's because it sought you out...and you agreed to it. You also looked for it, and you said yes to it.

Now, I am going to contradict myself. Saying yes is great but sometimes you need to say no, too.

When I first started Stella Jamieson Designs, I was selling my earrings at a local artisan vendor market. Approximately 30 other artists like myself were offering their goods there.

I was ecstatic because I thought it meant I would merchandise my earrings and reach more people with my craft.

My goal with every pair of earrings is to make people smile. They are meant to be fun and beautiful displays of art that you get to wear.

During the first month I spent at the shop, sales went well. It was summertime and tourists were visiting. However, once fall kicked in, not only did sales decline, but they literally didn't exist. That wasn't what I had in mind...at all!.
I was paying rent for a space in this shop, and I wasn't even making enough to cover my costs.

I knew this was a risk when I signed the lease, but it was a risk I had been willing to take. After all, I did have a full-time job, and this was just a side hobby. Additionally, I was aware that it took time to establish oneself as an artist, and I wasn't going to turn into Picasso overnight.

Each month that went by I continued to pay my rent on the spot, while my earrings collected dust. Any time I received an email from the shop, my heart would stop beating in my chest as I always thought this would email was the one notifying me I'd made a sale.

But it would just turn out to be another monthly newsletter, or an email to welcome a new vendor to the shop.

Finally, when one year had passed and they asked me if I wanted to renew my lease, I had to say no.

I could give you 100 reasons why I said no.

It was costing me money.

I wasn't selling anything.

The store wasn't getting a lot of foot traffic, so I wasn't reaching my intended audience.

Every month that passed without even a single sale depleted my self-esteem.

Truthfully, it was a combination of all these reasons and a few others.

However, all this didn't matter. The important thing was that I didn't want to put my earrings in that store anymore so I said no, and that was okay.

When something is no longer serving you, it's okay to stop. Too often, we feel pressured to continue with commitments and obligations even though they don't function for us. I'm not saying you should give up on your responsibilities, but if they no longer serve you and your heart isn't there, you can say no, and you don't need to feel badly about your decision. If this is how you perceive your situation, the chances are you aren't giving it your all anyway, and that isn't fair to the person or business on the other side of the fence. You could prevent them from realizing their full potential because you're half committed to them. Peace out and move along.

I recognize this is easier said than done, but we all know, making decisions is hard.

I had been enrolled in a program to help with my anxiety and I was deciding if I wanted to finish it or quit it. I had recently had to make a decision that at the end of the day wasn't a big deal but, living through the moment, I felt like I'd been asked to determine the fate of the world.

In reality, anxious Kylie would call ten people from a pre-determined list and explain the situation to them. She'd give them the pros, the cons, and her reasoning for why she wanted to quit. Then, she'd give them a set of ideas to oppose her arguments, and finally she'd ask them for their opinion.

Distressed Kylie couldn't turn to multiple people in this situation because she'd said something in one of the sessions that she found embarrassing. Because of this, she trusted only one person to help her make a decision. When something humiliating happens we just want to run away from it. Who wants to live through something embarrassing and then call up 10 people and tell them about it?

I'd rather have my weekly pay cut in half!

I only trusted one person. I went through my regular process with them, and we made a decision. It was at this moment that I had a sudden realization.

This individual I trusted wasn't any smarter on this topic than I was and didn't have any more information than I did. In fact, I knew more, because I had lived through this situation. This individual couldn't truly understand my feelings or the benefits the program was having on me. This individual only knew what I told them, and although I tried to draw a complete picture for them to understand my difficulties, it was still different than them actually living it in my shoes.

Even if this individual had been enrolled in the program with me and witnessed my embarrassing moment, he'd have experienced it differently than I had. Heck, he might have experienced the embarrassing moment himself, and he would have faced it differently.

Knowing this person wouldn't fully see things from my perspective, made me realize that nobody was more informed about my life's decisions, than I was. This reinforced for me the importance of trusting my gut and my choices without seeking external validation from others who couldn't possibly understand the logic and emotions behind my opinions at the level that I experienced them by living through them.

If I want to say no to an opportunity, I'm going to damn well say no. People can comment whatever they want as a result. They can speculate on why I made my decision or they can make up rumours, but none of it matters because I'm the one who needs to live with the consequences of my choices.

Come on guys, saying no can be therapeutic! Heck, how often do we go to events or agree to babysit for a friend even though it means we'll lose our chance to sleep in for the first time in 14 weeks? Too often!

Sometimes, saying no to a person, opportunity, or event means saying yes to yourself. There's nothing wrong with that!

There're many ways you can show up for yourself:
- Stand up for yourself.

- Treat yourself like you would treat a friend – you'd never tear your friend down with words the way you do it to yourself.
- Speak to yourself with kindness.
- Stop caring about what others think. As the saying goes, their opinion of you is none of your business.
- Let yourself feel your emotions and really acknowledge them.
- Stick to your boundaries.
- Chase your dreams.
- Make time for activities that bring you joy.

How are you going to show up for yourself?

What dreams are you going to actively chase?

Write 5 kind things you want to say to yourself, but as though you were talking to a friend.

"Self-care to me is doing something that brings me joy
and makes me feel good.
This becomes particularly useful on those days when
nothing feels good.
Self-care is making sure that your cup is full."

Kristy

3

Loving it up, and Feeling Good

Written with kindness by Kristy

Self-care to me is doing something that brings me joy and makes me feel good.

This becomes particularly useful during those days when nothing feels good. Self-care is about making sure that your cup is full.

Let's talk for a minute about what happens when you aren't taking care of yourself.

You begin to feel run down, agitated, exhausted, and maybe even reaching the point of experiencing burn out. These types of emotions are low vibrational. We can't attract good things into our life when we're in these types of states. Like attracts like. When you feel like garbage and you're upset, you bring more of that into your life.

When I was in a piss ass mood because I'd pushed myself or I'd done too much for others without giving myself time to recuperate, I just plummeted into a downward spiral. I was vicious to myself, and I'd allow the negative criticism to reign loud and proud. I permitted it to the point where I was in bed in tears, and asking myself what the damn point of it was.

By being in this habitual pattern, I attracted a lot of horrible things into my life. I had constant fights with people around me and doors were being closed because my thoughts and attitudes were negative toward everything. I felt unworthy of everything, so I gave up. If I thought of a bad moment, it amplified into a whole day, then a whole week. Life sucked and it continued sucking.

These situations happen when we push ourselves to a breaking point. When I reached that point, I allowed the most horrible thoughts to come to the surface. Then, I'd push them aside and neglect what my body needed - which was for me to slow down and take care.

Think about the type of life you attract when you're not taking care of yourself.

This is how mine looked.

I was lonely because I pushed my companions away. I had one friend I'd spend time with and I could see the resentment forming because I treated her poorly. I made everyone else think they were wrong, and I was convinced that they were purposely hurting me. I'd blame my friend for the way I felt — it was her fault I was stressed out and run down. Even though I was the one who worked on university homework 24/7. I got myself worked up over big assignments, and I wouldn't take any breaks. I was the one not taking care of myself; not allowing myself to breathe.

I was constantly set off by things other people said. I was reactive instead of responsive. When I pushed people away, I only isolated myself, and it made me feel more unworthy. I used to get so agitated by what came out of people's mouths, that I convinced myself I was the one who was hated by everyone. In truth, I was treating myself with hate and I wouldn't ease up.

I obsessively spent every moment I had thinking and talking badly about myself.

Everything that was happening I blamed on the fact that I couldn't do things because of my stress level. I refused to do social activities and even a trip to a grocery store was too taxing. When I was run down, my anxiety and depression worsened because I made myself undeserving of joyful things. The longer I neglected myself care, the more negative energy I invited into my life. I wasn't feeling good or being in a state of joy, so I couldn't attract opportunities that I truly wanted.

Neglecting my self-care has taught me that it would lead to more hurt. It just brought more damage into my physical and mental life. The best way I can describe it is that you imagine for example, that you have an infection and you're refusing to take antibiotics. Your body and mind need time to decompress and recharge. When you neglect that, you're allowing that infection to spread and worsen.

What should we do then? Well, you need to turn it all around and commit to your wellbeing. Right now, I want you to think of a list of ten things that bring you joy and make you feel good. It could be something as simple as soaking your tired feet in a big bowl of warm water, or something as generous as going out and getting a massage. It also could be a 20-minute nap, a day's road trip, a 5-minute breath-work practice, or getting Starbucks. The most important part of this list is that these activities *BRING JOY* and *GOOD FEELINGS*. This is the key!

My Feeling Good List

1.

2.

3.

4.

5.

6.

7.

8.

9.

10.

Can you write down more than ten? Even better! Jot it all down in front of you, and now take a look at your list. I want you to commit to doing one thing from your list at least once a day to make sure that you are getting into that good vibe. I'd like you to be certain that your cup is full.

Showing up with our most amazing versions of ourselves creates a high vibe. When you think about how you want your day to go and the energy you would like to have; don't you think of it as being the best day ever, full of high vibe energy, enjoyable conversations, and meaningful connections? Wouldn't you like to get the absolute most out of your life every single day? You can't have that if you're exhausted and feeling in these low vibrational states.

Your body and mind are yours, my love, and you only have one opportunity to live your life to the fullest. You'll need to do what it takes to take care of you and your precious life. It's up to you, and you alone.

I know this sounds scary, but honestly, to have that type of control over your life should give you a sense of power.

Now, sometimes it takes scheduling of self-care moments on your calendar to actually ensure you are making the time.

It **must** become a priority. Your mental health depends on it, and if you don't take care of yourself then who will?

This is an example of what my self-care looks like:

- *Yoga & gentle stretching 10 minutes a day.*
- *Getting one of my favorite beverages: Iced Chai Tea Latte, matcha*

Latte, or a good loose leaf breakfast tea with frothy oat milk to top it off.

- *Reading a book that will level up my self-development (It can be a physical book or audio book)*
- *Reading a fiction story. Sometimes it's nice to escape to a made-up world for a chapter or two.*
- *Getting outside. Go for a hike, a walk, sit on a beach, or sit in your garden.*
- *It doesn't matter where, but being outside in fresh air revitalizes the soul.*
- *Playing high vibe music! Singing at the top of your lungs or dancing moves the energy and puts me in a better state of being.*
- *My plants and gardening. I love tending to my lush and green Pothos plants. They brighten my spirits, and I just love getting soaked into their beauty.*
- *Anything where I'm being pampered such as getting a massage, a manicure and pedicure, having my lashes lifted and tinted, or even doing an at home sheet mask facial. This stuff makes me feel so damn good!*
- *Eating at least one nutritious meal a day. Eating nourishing food sends signals to our body that we look after and care for it. Hey, it can be*

hard to break old habits, but starting small can make it much easier.

- *Quiet time. Having time to be by yourself and to do whatever you want in that moment can make a world of difference for your soul. This can be anything from 15 minutes to a couple of hours as long as you can manage it. I aim to find 1 full hour for myself each day. Just work with the time you have and try to slip this 'me moment' into your daily routine.*

I want you to choose things that really make you feel good. I'm talking about feeling it within your core, in your soul, not just at a surface level.

Yoga has done that for me. When I'm in my class, it is honestly an outlet for me. I can move, stretch, and open up. I shift the stagnant and stuck energy around to get rid of it, and to make room for all the good energy I want to bring in. Feeling good is the goal. We want to feel good every single day. Prioritizing our self-care is going to help us achieve that.

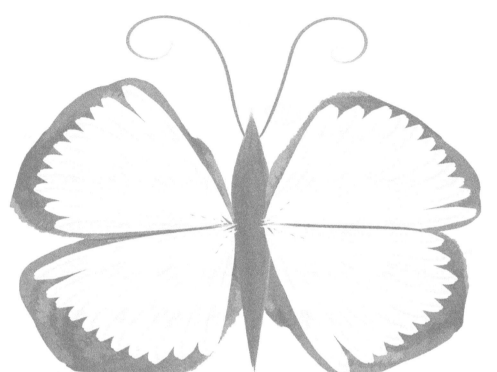

"When your attitude is gratitude, you open yourself up
to thinking of solutions
and problem-solving as opposed to creating more inner
turmoil for yourself."

Kristy

4

Observe First and Your Wings Will Come

Written with understanding by Kristy

Have you ever had a day when you've been all worked up because of something that what was coming? You didn't know how something was going to go, but you had already convinced yourself it wasn't going to go well? You saw a friend on Instagram who was spending their week exploring Scotland and you wished you were there instead of having to deal with your reality?

Your days begins. With anxiety already brewing, you're immediately hit with a conflict. Your gas light is on, so the tank is almost empty which means that you're going to be late. Someone begins to disagree with you as soon as you walk through the door of your office. You spill your tea all over some pretty important papers. Then, you have a very unpleasant encounter with a demanding person that you can't seem to escape, and you feel the verbal attack so deeply that you're trying not to explode. Bonus, you haven't charged your cell so it's about to die leading you to being unable to escape life for a few precious moments on social media. You feel overwhelmed by being hit with all this in an 8-hour span so you go home and stew about how wrong this day has gone. Your bad mood continues through dinner and maybe you even spill the food that you've just cooked, all over the floor! On your way to bed you realize that your laundry isn't done, and you're out of underwear for the rest of the week. Now, you're staying up late to finish at least one load, before getting an unrestorative sleep because your brain is still replaying every event from this horrible day.

Woah! That's a lot. Anyone else stressed just reading that? Okay, so before we go any further, I'm sure you can relate to those bad days just going to shit as they progress. Right?

Can I ask you a question? Do you believe that you actually create your day? It's quite possible you answered 'no', because if that was the case, why would most days be absolutely awful and feel like a struggle then?

Here is what I've come to learn. When we first become the observer of our thoughts, actions, and emotions, we begin to see what kind of part we play in our life's journey.

Let's begin with looking at the story above. Was it really that bad? In my experience of being an observer of this scenario, it wasn't the story that was terrible, it was the way the narrator told it. Don't get me wrong, I'm not putting any blame on the person experiencing these events. What I am saying is that we should take responsibility for our thoughts and actions.

What do we find when we look at this narrative of a really shitty day? Well, I'd say we have about 10 examples of where there were some unfortunate things that happened. During this bad day, there were times of conflict and discomfort; however, did all these things really sum up to a bad day? In a span of 24 hours these 10 conflicts seem pretty minimal in the grand scheme. Could it be possible that you actually had a neutral or a good day, but with a few bumps?

I want to look at this day from three different perspectives now. First, I will break it down on a scale:

- Friend in Scotland — upset and envious for 30 seconds-1 minute of scrolling.
- Empty tank of gas — annoyed and feeling rushed — 7 minutes to find a gas station and pump the gas.
- Being late to your job, meeting, school — wherever you're going — rushed and anxious —15 minutes late.
- Person confronting you about your lateness and starting a disagreement — overwhelming and anxious — 5-10 minutes
- Spilling your tea — annoying and an embarrassment — 6-minute clean up.
- Another person completely freaks out on you placing blame — 7

minutes of a verbally aggressive conversation.

- Cell phone dying — pissed off and feeling drained — 1-minute tops to realize you need to find a charger.
- Drop dinner on the floor — total annoyance (5-second rule! Just kidding!) 3-minute cleanup.
- Laundry — exhausted — 1 hour for washing and loading the dryer.

Not including the torturous thoughts you have spent reliving the day resulting in a restless night, we have a total of 1 hour and 50 minutes. Out of the entire day you've had, 1 hour and 50 minutes was spent within a negative emotion pattern, but you choose to write the whole thing off as a bad day in its entirety.

Do you notice how I've attached one or more emotions to each incident? The vibrations that you connect with in each occurrence is what makes the incident linger and feel longer than it actually was. This is one way to observe the thoughts on an after-math scale to put the day into perspective.

Can you see now how you create your day? You've labeled it a bad day and you've felt it emotionally as a bad day, even after the incident that had occurred is over. You've dwelt on it and made it even worse than it was, and you've allowed it to affect your evening, dinner as well as your sleep.

When you go on these downward spirals, take a pen and a piece of paper, and start writing about the event(s) of the day. I want you to look at the emotions you are giving them, what you are fixating on, and why it triggers you so much. Were you made to feel wrong? Were you embarrassed because of how you acted or reacted? Write it all down, don't place blame, but rather take responsibility for your behavior. Taking ownership will allow you to let these events go, because you've given yourself the power back.

Observe, observe, observe.

Stop associating these events with negative things within you or within others. If you need to scale it like we did above, it'll show in the grander vision of the day just how insignificant it really was.

Another way to observe this situation is to be a true viewer in *THE MO-MENT*. Let's look at the story again, but this time with an absolute neutral state of mind. This can take some practice, but here we go. Same scenario, staying neutral!

You wake up, it's just a normal day, and you get ready to go out. Your Instagram friend is exploring Scotland this week, you think that's amazing and you're happy for them.

You're driving your car and your gas gauge indicates that your tank is almost empty; you decide you'd better get some gas. The line at the gas station isn't very long, but it's possible you'll arrive late to your destination. Well, all you can do is prioritize your needs and know having enough gas will get you to your destination safely. You walk in the office door and someone points out that you are late, and disagrees with your explanation. They don't seem to want to hear it, so you simply allow them to accept what they wish knowing you have done your best. Later, you take out some papers but you turn too quickly, and you tip over your tea. You promptly do the only logical thing and clean it up, after all getting upset won't undo the spill. Later, a person confronts you aggressively and you calmly listen to what they have to say, accepting what they're telling you, and taking whatever responsibility you can to fix the problem they have expressed. Perhaps you ask them to come back when they feel calmer and less defensive so you can establish a resolution without any aggression. You go to check your cell and realize that you don't have a lot of battery left, so you ask someone to lend you a charger, and they do. Now, you can charge your phone without worrying about going without it, until you get back home.

When you finally get home, you aren't stewing over the day, but you're relaxing and enjoying watching your favorite sitcom as you begin cooking dinner. Again, you move too quickly, and the food falls on the floor. You act fast and scoop it up because, well, 5-second rule is a rule after all, (for real this time), and you proceed eat your dinner while enjoying a pleasant evening. When it's your bedtime you suddenly realize that you've run out of clean underwear. You grab a load and shove it in the washer, which is a great excuse to watch another episode of your sitcom while you wait for the cycle to finish so you can put the clothes in the dryer. Then, you go to bed not feeling anything negative about the events of the day, as it's been pretty uneventful overall.

Can you recognize the different feelings and vibration this day presented?

When we don't give any energy or negative emotion to the less than perfect events, they are just that, events. They're just incidents that have happened during the day but nothing that's worth reliving in our minds over and over. There wasn't any need to label it a bad day, because there wasn't any bad emotion that occurred. The day was just a day. We've created a neutral setting, and a neutrally emotional day's events in this story.

We're going to rewrite the story again but this time with emotions. These sentiments will be optimistic and we'll observe the day through a positive lens. We're going to watch our thoughts and actions in order to create a great day instead of a bad one. This one, like the neutral day, will take some practice. This technique may be one of the hardest ways to perceive your day. However, if you decide that it's easy to observe and you can redirect your thoughts to this method, then it'll be a natural progression for sure.

Here we go!

You're getting ready for your day and you take a moment to scroll through social media. You find out that your friend from Instagram is exploring Scotland this week, you think you might be jealous of them but when you really think of it, you'd rather spend a week in the Caribbean on a hot beach than in a rainy, cool country. In fact, you make a mental note that you'll be looking for some vacation destinations in the Caribbean this year.

You start the car and you see that the gas gauge shows the tank is almost empty.

You turn to gratitude and thanks for the 3 gas stations that are close to your house. You can stop at any of them before you reach your destination. You arrive 15 minutes late to your office as a result, and when you walk in someone points out how late you are. You try to explain but they just argue with you and don't want to hear what you have to say. You move on choosing to feel appreciated since they were expecting you, and you were missed.

Later, you sit down over some papers and because you move too quickly, you knock over your tea. You act fast and you grab something to mop the spill up with.

You're also relieved that you saved copy of the documents on your computer.

Later, you're stopped by someone confronting you aggressively, you ask them how you can support them, and you offer to find a solution together. By the end of the conversation, you have nothing but compassion for how upset and overwhelmed that person is, and you're grateful that you could help. You have a moment to check your phone and find it almost dead. You're thankful that you're around so many people, and you start asking if you can borrow someone's charger.

Obviously, someone has one to lend you.

In the afternoon you return home and you're excited to see that it's still nice outside, so you go for a walk. It's a peaceful and a great way to end your day. You come back home and you start making dinner, but moving too quickly you knock over the food, and it falls to the floor. You decide that you don't want to eat food from the floor, so you dispose of it. You're still feeling grateful because you have more ingredients left to make another meal.

You spend the rest of the evening winding down, but when it's bedtime you realize that you have no clean underwear for the next day. That's why you decide to stay up a bit longer to have one load of laundry washed. While waiting for the cycle to finish, you connect with one of your friends for a late-night chat to catch up. Finally, you put the clothes in the dryer and you go to bed, feeling grateful for the day you've had and ready for a restful sleep.

When your attitude is gratitude, you open yourself up to thinking of solutions and problem-solving, as opposed to creating more inner turmoil for yourself. While reflecting on these three ways of thinking, I want you, starting today, to observe your thoughts as you move through your day. Do your thoughts automatically go to negative and defensive thoughts? Can you switch them to a neutral thought or better yet, to a sense of gratitude? Your personal vibration attracts the same sentiments. Watch your thoughts, situations, and see how they affect your day.

We get to observe, revaluate, and redirect.

Perceive the why.

Be an observer of how you react to situations and to others. Be an observer of how others react to you. When we're in a state of 'reaction', there's something a little bit deeper there.

It can be formed by a past memory or an experience that we've allowed to be ingrained in us. Observing this can help you understand why you behave in certain situations the way you do. Then, you can come to heal it.

Here, I'd like to give an example of an event that has been trivial but significant to me. This is an observation that I've experienced.

Once upon a time, I was at university and I worked on a group project with one of my classmates. We were supposed to prepare an exhibition on the effects of fracking in rural communities and we found some horrific information, although that isn't what I was going to talk about. We'd both picked what we were going to present based on our collaborative collection of information and we were getting ready to show the final product.

A few days before our seminar which we were set to give a presentation for, we emailed each other back and forth going over final details. We noticed some missing information that could make for a lapse in the project. It was my responsibility to complete that part and it had completely slipped my mind. I'd honestly forgotten all about that data. When I explained this to my partner, they responded in this way, "I'm so sick of me pulling all the weight of my group projects, all you people are lazy, and you just want to get off with doing nothing. How could you forget about that?"

There I was in front of my computer, staring at that email, and bursting into tears. I felt so bad that I'd forgotten about collecting this information. I never wanted to be accused of trying to do less when I was striving to do my best, and working diligently to get my undergraduate degree. I had no words, I felt shame and embarrassment. I felt like I should drop out of school and return to my hometown to hide away from this mistake.

When you're already in a dark space, these types of situations can make you feel even worse. This event validated my feelings of unworthiness for getting my degree, and I felt that I should just give up. I beat myself up for weeks about this, even after I'd fixed my mistake and our presentation was given a grade of 87%.

Why did this person's statement shake me so deeply? This is where the observer side of me was completely absent. I took my project partner's remarks to heart, and I instantly believed them. I never questioned why she'd said that, or why I even accepted her remarks as truth. I didn't allow myself to take a step back and examine more deeply what was actually going on.

If I had become the observer, this would have been a totally different scenario. Let's take a glimpse at what this could have looked like.

The moment I received the email, if I had observed my reaction, I'd have been able to switch it to a response. The email stated, "I'm so sick of me pulling all the weight of my group projects, all you people are lazy, and you just want to get off with doing nothing. How could you forget about that?"

Instead of allowing myself to take those painful things in, as a part of who I was, I could have realized a couple of different things. First, I'd been hurt in the past by people saying cruel things to me, and I'd allowed myself to expect and accept that these comments were real. When I knew deep in my heart that it wasn't the truth, my story about myself mimicked the one my project partner had told. If I were to look at the reality that was right in front of me, I'd see the truth about who I really was.

I was a 20-year-old woman taking five university classes, all with full time workloads of projects, tests, term papers, presentations, seminars, labs, and lectures. I was working my ass off during late nights, spending weekends in the library, barely eating, isolating, and making myself physically sick. I'd wake up at 3:00 a.m. and throw my guts into the toilet because of stress and worry.

Despite all of that, I was doing my absolute best. You need to know that these years of my late teens/early twenties were a really dark place for me. However, if I had this particular tool of being an observer at that time, everything would have changed. This being said, I'm glad I have it now so I can reflect on this moment and question the truth. Back to my memories: I was a stressed-out university student, overworked, and not taking care of herself.

No wonder I accepted my project partner's words so readily, although I wasn't in a good state to take these words in or to process them fully at the time. Instead, I just agreed that I was probably lazy like everyone else, and I probably didn't want to do any work. Even though, in reality I was in the same boat as my classmate with other assignments, while my group members were completely M.I.A.

If I'd taken a step back, I'd have been able to process what was happening outside of myself more effectively. I could have seen what was taking place on her end, which ironically was also happening to me. I could have had compassion and seen the stress that she was feeling on her end. I could have recognized myself in her. She was obviously feeling pressure to get through her schoolwork and to hold up her end of the group assignment. She also might not be taking care of herself the way she should, just like I wasn't. Her email literally screamed "I AM SOO FRUSTRATED AND DEFEATED."

If I'd been the observer of the thoughts that came up, I'd have recognized that I wasn't a lazy person, but quite the opposite. I wasn't trying to get out of the workload, I genuinely forgot to do my share, and with everything I was juggling, it was really obvious how that had happened. I could have also shown compassion to myself and to my classmate. She was going through similar stresses that I was experiencing. Instead of apologizing and accepting her words, I could have said, "I want to express regret for forgetting about this point. I will rectify it before our presentation. I also want to say that I'm far from lazy or trying to get you to do more work than we've agreed on. I understand the importance of the project, and I also understand the stress that university life brings. Please know that my grades matter to me, and I wouldn't try to jeopardize them on purpose. Is there anything else that I can help with to get done apart from getting the information to complete our presentation?"

Had I said that, I'd be able to come from the energy of calmness and neutrality, and I would have been able to respond instead of react or blame myself and her.

Seeing ourselves in other people may allow us to understand what is really going on, and that has nothing to do with you. My classmate's reactive email had nothing to do with me. This had been what she had been feeling, and she was projecting it onto me, because she needed to blame someone. In my experience when people begin to be rude, defensive, or standoffish it's because something deeper is going on in their world. How do I know this? Because I see myself in them, that is exactly how I used to react in the past and I still do sometimes.

A few months ago, I worked at a retirement home. Each day was busy with all the daily ins and outs of the home, ensuring our residents were happy, verifying that the protocols for the COVID-19 regulations set out by the government were being followed, answering questions to families about how to better care and protect their loved ones from the virus, and so much more. One week, we'd gotten swamped with new mandates, and we were setting up our home to follow the protocols precisely.

Before I knew it, it was Friday and I just finished helping our team get everything in order for the mandate deadline. I was stressed, exhausted, my head was pounding, and I had forgotten to eat lunch. One of my coworkers came up to me and asked if I'd ordered their new mop because the order arrived and it wasn't there. At this point, I snapped. I felt like nobody had any idea what I'd been through. They obviously didn't see me running around like a chicken with its head cut off! I reacted like this, "No, I didn't because I forgot about it, and someone could have reminded me to order all the things. Sometimes I can't just drop everything and do what you want. I've been running crazy trying to help get the mandates in order rather than worrying about a mop."

I lashed out at my co-worker and they matched my tone. "Fine, I will ask someone else!" This fired me up even more, because I felt they were questioning my ability to do the job. I let it go and went home for the weekend. I stewed about it all Friday night until I went to bed. The next morning, I woke up as the observer. Now that I was well-rested, and I had time to rethink the whole situation, I could see what was going on. I forgot to do a task that was just as important as the mandates. They needed that mop. I let myself get so stressed out that I was overlooking the small things. After deliberating I took responsibility for my actions, I was again not taking care of my wellbeing and allowing my reactiveness to control the situation. I let my insecure self come through and feel threatened so much that I was rude and defensive towards my co-worker, who just came to ask a simple question.

On Monday, I apologized to my co-worker. I said that I'd been pushing myself and felt horrible that I'd let them down on getting the correct supplies. I felt possessive about my job and I couldn't admit that having someone else help me out would be nice. It was because at that time I thought it was them simply saying that I couldn't do my job, or that I wasn't good at it.

I made these stories sound real, but they weren't true. When I observed the situation afterwards, I could see my reaction for exactly what it was, an insecure story I used to have about myself that had crept back into my mind when I was in a low vibration.

It still happens sometimes that I forget to be the observer of the situations, and it takes me back to an anxious place immediately.

This is an interesting topic, so let's continue even deeper now. Let's look at being an observer of just your thoughts. Not the thoughts that come about when a situation happens, or you get triggered, but just everyday thoughts that you have about yourself and maybe someone else.

As an observer, we're neutral to our thoughts, allowing them to come and steer us towards different situations. When these thoughts appear, I want you to label them as either low vibe or high vibe. Low vibe thoughts are the negative and judgmental ones, the ones where you're in the middle of something, you're putting yourself down, and speaking poorly in your mind about yourself. Please categorize your perceptions and keep a tally of how many thoughts are high vibe or low vibe.

When I first started doing this, my low vibe thoughts outnumbered my high vibe thoughts. That's absolutely okay, because the point of this exercise is to observe and to become aware.

Day 1

Vibrational Tally

<————————————>

High vibe thoughts   Low vibe thoughts

For someone with anxiety, I probably had 10 high vibe thoughts to every 100 low vibe ones. As you can tell, my mind sought out judgment, negativity, and self-sabotaging over love, happiness, and gratitude that could render you into a high vibration.

Now, please remember I'm not saying this to create more work for you or to have you adding many things to the to-do list, but to become aware. You can keep a tally or as you go through your day, just take a mental inventory.

You may even start your day and before you leave your house, you already have a general consensus of what vibe occupies your thoughts. Please don't become judgemental if your list is composed, like me, of many low vibe thoughts. There isn't any wrong here, we're simply observing.

Once you've gotten the idea of what thoughts are dominating your mind, let's start Day 2 activity.

Day 2

This one may take persistence and willpower, so I want you to be diligent in it.

This is where taking your power back begins. Each time a low vibe thought rears its ugly head, I want you to question it almost as if you are undermining it.

Ask the following questions:

But what if this was different?

Is this actually the truth?

Is this a story that I tell myself?

Do I choose to believe this thought?

Why am I believing this thought?

Is this thought a fear-based thought?

Questioning the low vibe thoughts slowly takes their powers away. It allows the brain to evaluate which ideas you want to take on and which you don't. You can do the same for the high vibe thoughts.

Ask the following questions:

This is good, but how can I think even greater?

Could this be elevated by x, y, z?

Is this thinking small?

What could make me feel even more abundant right now?

Elevate your thoughts because, if you've noticed, your thoughts become your reality. Okay, you spent time questioning those low vibe voices that live in your head. So what?

Well, before we move on, I want to ensure that you consistently practice the questioning. It doesn't stop. The moment we stop questioning the thoughts, you give your power back to the thought rampage. Do yourself a favor, and master this.

Day 3

This is a Day 3 exercise. After you've gotten into the habit of questioning your perceptions, the next step is to replace them with love based and good feeling thoughts.

Here is an example of what my inner dialogue was like in my darkest, anxiety ridden moments.

Ugh, another day of stress and exhaustion.

I'm already late, and the presentation I've got today made me so worried that I didn't sleep. I'm so tired. I'm probably going to fail, anyway. Ugh, I do everything wrong and I'm the worst student. I feel too sick to eat.

I'll probably miss the bus. I look like shit; I feel like shit. How can anyone love me? No wonder I have no friends. Oh my god, it's so cold outside and I just want to go back to bed. I have no energy. I hate my life. Why is that girl telling her life story at the top of her lungs on the phone on the bus? It's too early to deal with this. What is that person wearing? It looks like a Halloween costume. This seat on the bus makes me so carsick. The person next to me reeks of cigarettes. My stress is starting to rise. I feel like I may be sick. That woman is so beautiful!

I look like a toad next to her. I hate my stupid self. I should really go to the gym. Why am I not prettier? I could be fitter. I hope my professor doesn't call on me today.

I wonder if it's even worth it to walk to class. I'm going to fail everything, anyway.

I always do. I just want to disappear. Nobody would miss me. I'm a burden, anyway. I annoy my boyfriend; I think he's just with me because I'm pathetic, and he feels sorry for me.

He wouldn't miss me. I spent all this money on school, and I'm nothing but a screw up. I'm such a failure. I'm worthless. I just pray to a God I don't believe in that the teacher won't call on me to participate in the lecture. I feel sick again. Oh God, my hands are shaking, my heart is going to burst out of my chest. My mouth is so dry I feel like I'm going to die right here in class.

I don't want to die. I feel dizzy. The teacher calls on me. I know the answer is right here in my notes, yet I utter, "I don't know." Why did I say that? She asks if I did the reading assignment. I feel my extremities going numb. "I did", I answer. Why is she singling me out? I'm about to die right in front of her. I read off my page. Ugh, my voice is so shaky. "Sustainable development."

I can't breathe! She says 'correct' and moves on through the lecture. I'm such an idiot. How embarrassing. Everyone thinks I'm a loser now.

This snapshot is just within a few hours of my morning, not even the whole day. I wished I had known then what I know now. But here we are. Doing a little tally, you can see that the majority of my thoughts (if not all) were low vibrational. Does anyone feel icky just reading all that?

Doing the exercise from Day 2 would have shown how my thinking patterns were based on fear-based thoughts.

Here come the questions:

But what if it was different?

What if it didn't have to be another day of stress and exhaustion? What if it was easy and neutral?

What if I wasn't late? What if everything was in divine timing?

Is this the truth?

Was I actually failing? Did I actually feel like shit? Do I actually look like shit? Do I really have no friends? Do I really hate my life?

Is this a story that I tell myself?

Is this the same narrative that I used yesterday? Everyday?

Am I narrating my life all based on fear?

Do I choose to believe this thought?

I'm choosing to believe that it's a crappy day. I'm choosing to think that I hate myself and I'm a failure. I'm choosing to allow these thoughts to make me physically sick. I'm also letting these perceptions convince me I'm stupid, worthless, and unloved.

Why am I believing this thought?

I believe it because I've persuaded myself it's true. It's habitual, and it's becoming instinctive.

It seems easier to think in fear than to push for love.

Is this a fear-based thought?

Yes, I've lived with these thoughts for so long that my mind has gotten accustomed to them.

It's an automatic thought reel that replays each day, and I've never thought any different.

It's always been my normal reaction to everything that's been happening.

Let's take a minute to really think about this. Pretend you live with a roommate who does nothing but say these things to you. They put you down, tell you they hate you, and they think you're a stupid, worthless failure. You'll never be pretty enough. You should just die because no one cares enough to miss you, anyway. Your life sucks as you're a fat, exhausted, sickly person.

These kinds of thoughts in your head are basically like having a toxic roommate. Except with an actual roommate, I'd hope I had the strength to evict them or to move out. However, the toxic roommate in your head is just allowed to be there, and they make you believe in every word they say. My love, it's high time to get rid of that roommate!

Exercises

Observe the thought, question the thought, and replace it. Every time a low vibe thought comes up, we're going to stop it in its tracks. You can literally hold your hand up and say firmly, "NO, I choose something different!"

We'll go back to my low vibe thought monologue now. Let's replace our perceptions!

- Instead of stress and exhaustion, I choose ease and an energizing day.
- Instead of being tired and seeing myself as a failure, I'll question. I know for a fact that I've succeeded in everything I've done, and I feel so good about that. I'm a rockstar!
- Instead of not eating, I'll bring snacks because I'll get hungry.
- Instead of being a horrible student and being late, I decide that I'm a perfect student and an adult who can own up to their lateness. I also deserve my extra sleep and if I miss the bus, there will be another one in 10 minutes.
- Instead of putting myself down about the way I look and blaming that on the fact that I have no friends, I question that thought and I choose differently. The truth is that:
- I'm beautiful just the way I look. It doesn't matter if I go to the gym or put make-up on, I'm beautiful. One more thing, I have so many

amazing friends who love and support me and a boyfriend who adores me.

- Instead of thoughts of judgment towards other people, I choose loving thoughts.
- That woman is so passionate about what she's saying. I really want to harness that kind of conviction when I speak. That beautiful woman has inspired me to try a new make-up routine.
- Instead of anticipating thoughts about being called on or screwing up, I choose to believe in myself. I'm a good student in my own way. I have the answers and my teacher knows it. That's why she always calls on me. I'm determined to trust that there isn't any way I can ruin anything. I can only learn.
- Instead of caring what other people think of me, I choose to love myself. If I get a little hung up on words as I talk, that's okay. I'm learning to speak in public as I hope to travel and give a speech one day.

At first, this may seem a little difficult, but with time, it becomes so much easier. The kinder and more emphasis on the "EXTRA LOVE", the better. Talking gently to yourself creates a new reality for you. For me, it's built a reality of love for myself and others, friendship, opportunity, chasing my dreams (and I have big ones), freedom, and true happiness.

I want you to know this. I HATED myself so much that I was considering

dying as a viable option. As I'm typing these words now, there're so many emotions coming to the surface. Through observing my thoughts, not only could I change them, but I also forgave myself and began to love myself. It all must come from you.

The only suffering we endure is the suffering we impose on ourselves repeatedly.

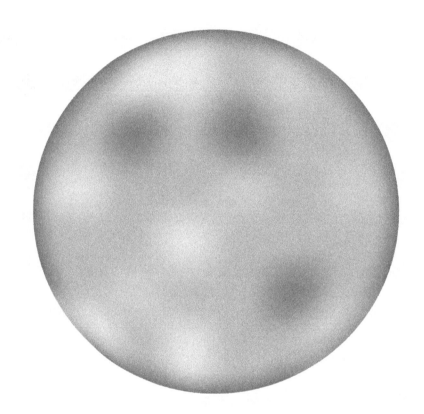

"Are we even truly living?"

Kylie

5

The Reason Within Your Wings

Written with desire by Kylie

When you think of purpose, what is the first thing that comes to your mind? For me, it used to be the 2015 album *Purpose* by Justin Bieber. Even now, I can hear the sweet melody of his soft voice flowing through my brain as I recall the lyrics to one of his songs, ***"Sorry"***.

I was attending Carleton University when this album was released, and I can recall how crazy the sorority girls would get at a fraternity mixer when this song was played.

Now that I have aged... not quite like a fine wine, but more like cheese perhaps. Purpose means something different to me. Of course, I still hum JB's tunes, but there's more depth to it than there used to be.

There are two parts to purpose: intention and reason. Let's break this down!

Intention

When something is done intentionally, you're actively thinking about what you're doing. It isn't like the car ride to work where you get there and wonder how the heck you made it, because you were lost in your thoughts and now you don't recall the drive. You're actively engaged in the process from start to finish. You have the thought of what actions you need to take, and then you take those actions with full awareness while you're doing it.

Reason

The reason is your why. It's what fuels you and what drives you. It's what inspires you, motivates you, and captivates you. It's the feeling bubbling within you, calling you to engage in certain activities in order to fuel this fire.

Okay, Kylie and Kristy, this is all great, but how do I discover my purpose?

Grab a piece of paper and a pen. Find a cozy chair. Now, write down every area of your life.

This is what my list looks like:

Business

Chaos & Bliss Poetry

Exercise

Working on a book with Kristy

Volunteer

Work

Friends

Family

Animals

Make sure you include everything. It may help to let the list sit for a bit and then come back to it to see if there're any areas you might have forgotten about. I actually keep my list posted on my desk so I can look at it every day. It helps me determine what I need to focus on during a particular day.

Once you have your list, attach feelings to each area. Do you feel full of life when engaging in any of the activities? Do you feel stressed? Do you feel bored? It's your decision if you want to label the areas as GOOD vibes or BAD vibes, or specify which emotions you feel about each of them. Here is my list again:

Business — joy

Chaos & Bliss Poetry — joy, relief

Exercise — passion

Working on book with Kristy — excitement

Volunteer — fulfilled

Work — fulfilled

Friends — joy

Family — joy

Animals — love

Once you have your list completed, take a good, hard look at it. This is going to help you determine what areas of your life fill your cup. Certain parts can't obviously be avoided. For example, you need a job. However, working on your list might help you realize your job isn't serving you, and you might consider looking for a new one. Please be aware that not every part of your life will bring you joy. That's okay!

Think back to the chapter on **Becoming An Observer**. Perhaps the circumstances don't need to change, but your perspective on the situation does. I get annoyed at my day job sometimes. Who doesn't? But overall, it brings me a sense of accomplishment and I enjoy what I do.

Look at your list again, choose the parts that stand out, and write what feelings they bring.

I enjoy volunteering,

I find self-care important,

I enjoy most areas of my life,

I enjoy being creative,

I like to help others.

THIS is where you'll find your purpose. When you reflect on and evaluate the areas of your life and what fulfills you, you'll find your motivation. My aim in life is to use my creativity to help others. This is what fuels me, what drives me, and what motivates me to be a better person.

If you're struggling to find your purpose, you may not be making the right choices in your life. Therefore, it's important to try new activities. I used to be hard on myself because I'd try so many things, and then I felt like I was quitting a lot. My friend, Christine, told me she didn't view it as giving up. She was actually inspired by me trying new projects and she thought that this way I was learning what I wanted in life, and what wasn't serving me. Heck, I even signed up for a volunteer firefighter session one night!

If you're looking at your list and struggling to see your purpose in life, try something new. Try volunteering. Try crafting. Look for a new job. Teach yourself a new skill.

Ask yourself these questions:

What is something I have always wanted to try?

What situations do I leave feeling like my heart is full?

What social issues do I care about?

What changes would I like to see in the world?

Who inspires me? Why do they inspire me?

Once you've really drawn out your purpose in life, this is your reason for being.

Now, we need to concentrate on the intention. Actively take steps to ensure you are living your life on purpose, with purpose, and for purpose.

In my life, I take steps to ensure I exercise my creativity to help people. There're multiple examples of situations where I do that, and one of them is Co-Chair for the Staff Wellness Committee at my job. I work in Corrections, which is an environment that can be draining, negative, and toxic. I help staff focus on their wellbeing by utilizing my creativity to plan events that can take their minds away from the negative aspects of the job, and help them focus on positivity and comfort. This brings me joy and fills my cup.

When you think about your purpose, what steps can you take to make certain you're living a life aligned with your purpose? Once you discover your steps, actively engage in them. Another list I keep on my desk is a list of activities I can do to stay aligned with my purpose, such as writing and making earrings. This guarantees I always stay on track.

One day, I saw an image while scrolling through Instagram. There were people sitting on the subway. When I looked at this photo, I stopped scrolling and I felt pure terror. I thought about life and what its meaning was. All these people looked as if they were shuttled onto a bus going through the same motions.

You're born. You spend your childhood wanting to become an adult. Then, you spend your adulthood wishing you were a child again. You pay bills. You pay off debt. You seek promotions. You get 2 weeks of vacation a year. You work to pay off your house. Then you die. It made me think, "Are we even truly living and if we are, why? What drives us? What makes this all worthwhile?"

This can feel daunting. What a huge dilemma to figure out! That's why you need to discover your purpose in life, so that you could have a reason to exist and are not just going through the motions like a herd of cattle.

The title of this book is **Becoming A Butterfly**, and it was an obvious choice. Kristy and I didn't take long to deliberate on the title. It fit perfectly for us right from the beginning.

The message is that in order to become a butterfly; you have to be a caterpillar first. You need to step through and grow through the uncomfortable first, and then you become a beautiful, magical, and free butterfly.

During the transition from a caterpillar to a butterfly, the caterpillar is very clear on its purpose and the result is magic and beauty. You'll notice that the purpose of the caterpillar changes once it becomes a butterfly. That's okay! Your purpose can shift as you grow and become someone else. Embrace the difference. Be open to learning, experiencing, and exploring new things that add to your purpose. Become the butterfly!

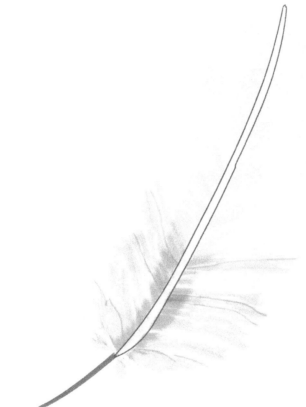

"I was born worthy. I do not have to prove myself;

I do not have to do anything at all to be worthy. I was

born worthy (and so were you)."

Kylie

6

Fly Butterfly, Fly

Written with peace by Kristy

Many years ago, I was on my reading week and going over my assignments that were given to me to complete after the break. I was overwhelmed. My anxiety and stress levels were at an all-time high. I doubted myself whether I could do a good job and stay focused. I felt I was going to fail everything. My brain seemed to work against me, unable to concentrate and making me constantly aware that I had so much to do before the week was out. Defeat was at the pinpoint of my mind.

My Facebook Messenger went off. My friend texted me saying she was feeling the same way. She wrote, "I'm not being productive. I haven't even broken 1000 words yet. I'm looking at the work pile and getting discouraged."

I, immediately forgetting my stress, said. "It's okay. Maybe take a break, make some tea, get some brain food, and step back from it instead of forcing it. You can take the rest of the evening off. We still have 6 days before its due date."

She replied, "I've got the tea and I've just made dinner with a friend. I'm just stressed because I feel like I haven't done anything this evening. I'm not getting anything done."

I suggested she started again tomorrow, and she decided to go to the library the following day. My mood changed after I'd helped her find her way through it.

I also could see that I was ready and available to be there for my friend, believing in her ability to do the assignments and be okay, but I wasn't doing the same for myself.

Could I not be my own best friend? Why couldn't I be there for myself and believe in myself? I always trusted in everyone else. When there was something I wanted to do, but I believed I couldn't, I would suggest it to someone I thought was more capable (usually my younger sister).

In high school, I told her she should join the volleyball team. I wanted to do this myself, but felt I couldn't. I didn't believe in me, Kristy. At university, when it came to applying for summer jobs, I would encourage my friends to go for the position that would give them experience in their field. I only applied for jobs that would just get me a job. I never dared to even try. I didn't believe I could. I didn't believe I was worthy enough.

I wanted so badly to study abroad in England, Scotland, or another European country. When it came to applying for it, I backed out because I got anxious about going. I didn't think that I could go abroad, live there, take care of myself, and be okay. I didn't believe in my confidence to do something that "extreme". Many friends and my sister took that leap and had amazing adventures. I was mad at myself. I was missing out because my anxiety was feeding me false stories of unworthiness and doubt. I trusted that everyone else could do anything they wanted, but I didn't have that faith in myself.

What was going on with me was this: I didn't believe in myself because of what I believed about myself.

What was I believing about myself?

I believed *I was unworthy.*
I believed *I was broken.*
I believed *I was unloved.*
I believed *I was ugly.*
I believed *I couldn't do anything.*
I believed *I was a poor student that ended up at university by some mistake.*
I believe *I wasn't smart.*
I believed *I wasn't confident.*
I believed *I wasn't able.*
I believed life would *be better without me.*

90

I believed *I was worthless*.

Now that I'm looking at all these self-beliefs, I'm not surprised I never did anything outside my comfort zone. As I got older and leaned more into these types of assumptions, I continued to put off more adventures, more opportunities, and isolate myself.

These beliefs made me lead a life of anger, where I was blaming others for my misery.

I was agitated, annoyed, and reactive to all the things that made me feel anxious, from the time I woke up in the morning till the thoughts that stayed with me while I was falling asleep.

Over time, I grew to understand that I was the one causing all this to happen. It wasn't other people that were making me feel this way; it was me. I believed these perceptions about myself, what in result rendered them true. They became my reality. Unworthiness I was feeling affected my thinking and behaving in such ways, that I perceived everything around me as the evidence of that state.

Only recently (almost 7 years later), I started to recognize these beliefs and began to shift and change them.

I no longer wished to live in fear or in lack, so I chose new feelings. I wanted to start my own online yoga business and in order to do that, I couldn't keep the perceptions I previously had. No, they needed to transform.

I wanted to be a successful businesswoman. A successful businesswoman doesn't think she's unworthy. Without doubt, she believes in her worth and that she's enough. She perceives herself as intelligent, confident, beautiful, and more than able to accomplish her dreams. She is sure she can do things, and she trusts herself.

I knew what I had to do to become **HER**. I needed to direct my thoughts, feelings, and behavior to this successful version of myself. Since I could never achieve this change with my previous beliefs, I started to embody these new perceptions, and after a while, they stuck with me. From time to time, I still have that little voice step in and let me know how I can't do things, or how I'm not worthy. It's an old version of myself, and I can't let it back in.

The greatest part of my transformation is that I get to decide and be in control.

I'm choosing to believe in those images of myself that are empowering, make me feel strong, radiant, and bold. I no longer wish to go back to the beliefs that kept me hating my self-made miserable life, feeling isolated, and in low vibrational energy.

I started to define what these new perceptions looked like. Being successful meant to me running my own business. How could I appear as a prosperous person? I worked on it. I sent emails; I updated the content on social media, and I did some advertising. I taught regularly and with confidence.

Faith meant to me showing up despite nervousness, telling myself I've got this, and trying new things outside of my comfort zone. When I started doing scary things, they became less frightening. I fully stepped into that habit. I knew everything I needed to about teaching and I began doing it more often. I also started talking to people outside my social circle. I would chat with persons at the grocery store, on social media, and basically with anybody I met doing my daily activities. I started getting used to just having a simple conversation with people around me. As I did this, my confidence grew.

I could figure anything out, and this belief was pivotal. I no longer used excuses for why I couldn't deal with some business aspects. I just made everything work. I would search information on the internet, ask someone for help, or just go with the old, good trial and error. The only obstacles I had were the ones I put in front of me.

I was intelligent. I could truly think outside of the box and make things happen without getting discouraged, because they weren't going a particular way. I broadened my horizons so that I could become more efficient at problem solving. I believed that an intelligent woman wouldn't accept defeat when things went wrong, but she would look beyond the issue, reframe her perception of things, and incline to creative solutions. She would also learn and evolve, take all her knowledge and embody it.

I was born worthy. I didn't need to prove myself. In fact, I didn't need to do anything at all to be worthy. I was born worthy. And so were you!

Now I know that I'm not obliged to do anything special like moving mountains or making incredible discoveries. That's not what defines my worth. I'm worthy just as I am, and I'll never forget it.

Can you see this energy shift in redefining beliefs about myself? These perceptions make me feel more empowered and in control. They help me live the life that I want. I can take trips, meet, and connect with new people. I'm not afraid to go for those big dreams like writing this book, and I love life the way I was intended to.

Can I ask you something? What are you believing about yourself? Do you accept that you're nothing outside of your anxiety? Grab a pen and paper and take a few minutes to reflect on these questions.

What if you could make your dreams become reality? What would you be dreaming of?

Take a few moments to jot down a huge dream, nothing small. I'm talking about an ideal job, a big and explorative trip, or the best relationship ever! Whatever it may be, write it down on your paper to capture every last detail.

Fine! It can be something small, but make it something that excites you, okay?

Now that you have it all written down, I want you to examine all the reasons why you don't believe in yourself enough to accomplish your dreams. Bring up all the dirt here, leave nothing unburied. Dig it all up! Write down as much as you wish to.

Looking at your dream, think who you need to become to make it a reality. What beliefs do you need to shift to embody the person who would accomplish your dreams? Ask yourself if the perceptions you have about your right now match the image of that person. Write down how you need to change, what that means for you, and what opinions about your new self you're going to have.

Of course, once we've redefined our beliefs, it isn't enough to just write them down.

We must act the part! You've written about the embodiment of these new opinions, and now it's time to go out into the world and really live as this new you. "Strut your stuff", if you will.

What are you going to do to personify the idea of your new self in order to make it your reality? For example, if you're to make yourself accept that you're beautiful, you'll be practicing mirror work, telling yourself how beautiful your eyes, ears, nose, and hair are. (By the way, this practice won't take long for you to start believing it). Write it all down and if it becomes overwhelming, start with one belief, nurture it for a while, and then add some others.

These self-beliefs become crucial as we begin to build ourselves up to ultimately believe *IN* ourselves. Just watch how invincible you'll become. When you trust yourself, no one's perceptions about you or the world can penetrate your faith.

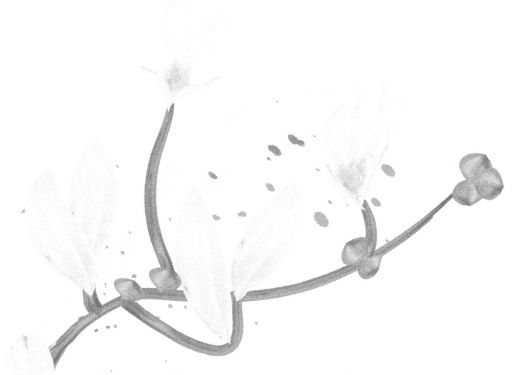

"We control our feelings, emotions, beliefs and actions from within, and our outside will mirror back to us as a match."

Kristy

Aligning With Your Butterfly

Written with tranquility by Kristy

In the chapter ***Fly Butterfly, Fly***, I asked you to write about a dream and then we looked at the beliefs you had around your vision. We saw how those perceptions would probably prevent you from getting from the place where you were at the moment to your desired dream. As a result, we revamped our opinions so that we could be a match with our desired self.

How is stepping into those beliefs coming along? Have you really been working on them? The thing is, Kylie and I can give you all the tips and tricks in the world, but we can't make the change for you. It must be you! You must want to do the inner work in order to build a better life!

As you can see from these chapters, Kylie and I have done the work. Am I saying it's easy? Well, if I'm being honest; if you want to change, then yes, it's simple. Try to compare your life at this moment, which might be in such a dark place, to what it could be. It could be filled with love and friendship, full of adventure and exploration, so incredible that when you go to sleep at night, you can't wait to wake up and start a new day.

To me, there was no competition. My life sucked, and my feelings shaped my attitude and behaviour. I was miserable, and I made damn sure that everyone around me felt the same way. I lived a life of judgment and gossip. This wasn't serving me because not only did I hurt others, but also myself. Talking poorly about other people did nothing for my energy, it just kept me in that low vibration. I judged myself even more, and I picked apart everything about me. I hated waking up and I would take naps to escape my daily life. I didn't want to admit that I was wrong. I never took ownership of things, and I could never be a leader.

I told you how I isolated myself, and I always picked petty fights with my friends.

I believed I was unlovable and I wouldn't achieve anything great or significant. I hated who I was, and I wished I was someone else. I felt trapped in a stupid, ugly body and if I was another person, my life would be astronomically better. I didn't bother having goals because, with the beliefs I had, I would never accomplish them.

I didn't think that I could possibly do well in life because I wasn't the smartest, the most popular, or the most beautiful. I felt like I always came in second and I lived in a world that was second best to my true calling and my true purpose. I was settling and accepting that my anxiety was the true determining factor. I lived in fear and I made myself dumb. I was embarrassed by everything I'd said to another person, and I felt that I'd be judged if I expressed myself or talked about my dreams.

Trying something new and out of my comfort zone kept me paralyzed and the thoughts "what if I fail" would affect my decisions. So, I stayed. I lived in fear and I was afraid of talking to people and trying new things. I just remained in the safety of my apartment where I didn't say anything that would embarrass me or call for judgment. I was alone, just me and my opinions that were driving me to suicidal thoughts. I could never break free from them, never question anything. I would only accept what I had. My life in my head was lonely and insignificant. I was a waste of breath and nobody could stand being near me. They would just tolerate me because they felt sorry for me. I convinced myself that I was a disappointment to my parents. My boyfriend didn't love me, and my siblings thought I was a big loser. I wasn't moving forward or growing; I was stagnant.

That reality, compared to the life I wanted, was a no brainer. Once I figured out that the only person who could give me that existence was me, I took control back. I felt invincible.

I wasn't going to let anyone tell me what I could or couldn't do, let alone my ego.

The beliefs I had about myself changed. They were empowering and transformative. When I saw how easily I could become the person I always desired to be, I kept progressing.

I started a yoga business, created an online studio and mindset courses, entered competitions, signed up with a coach, and I traveled to Mexico on the most luxurious vacation of my life.

I made the motions to do the things I wanted and now I'm writing a book. My goals have unfolded before my eyes.

Having goals gives us something to look forward to, to be in joyful expectation, and really see what we want out of our lives. It also helps us have that truly fulfilling existence.

Let's go back to your big dream! Write your big goal here:

This is what I want you to focus on. The bigger, the better, the more exciting (maybe a little scary), and the more you want it. I believe you can have anything you want in this life, so get unapologetic about it. There is no judgment here, and no dream is too big.

I'd suggest keeping the goal you've written above with you. You can use it as a background on your phone or put it down on a piece of paper that you'll carry in your pocket. This way, you can return to it regularly and keep it as the focus of your mind.

Now, I want you to write about all the ways this goal will affect you. Describe how it'll affect your life and the people around you. What will change if you reach this goal?

Write about all the whys. Why do you want this goal? Giving your objective a 'why' connects you to purpose, and it'll keep you from faltering from it.

Will it give you more money to be generous? (To family, to community, to charity) Will it get you on that cruise you've been searching for the past few months? Will you be of service or help someone? Will it be something you are passionate about? Why is this goal important to you? Remember, the more specific, the better.

The "why" allows you to focus a little deeper on what the goal is, and it gives you a reason to hold this objective at laser focus.

The next step is to take spiritually aligned action toward your goal. What does that mean? It means to become a match to your goal, just like we did with the beliefs. You can act all day long on your goal and you may see gradual results, or you may see no results at all. When we become this match to our goals, what does it mean? Well, it looks like this.

You should be in the energy of the goal you want to achieve and feel the excitement, pride, accomplishment, and joyful expectation. You never want to act toward your goal with the force of annoyance, forced action, anger, frustration, or exhaustion. The spirit you put there becomes your vibration of the product. Your thoughts, feelings, energy, and actions become your reality (remember the chapter on becoming an observer). I would say that it's like moving the needle forward.

That's not to say that the actions from your low vibrational state won't move you forward; however, your progress might feel slow and appear gradual. I'm speaking from experience when I tell you that when we feel the energy of the goal, it appears faster and without resistance.

One day, I wanted to test this theory of spiritually aligned action toward my goal.

On a random Wednesday, I set a target of making $1.000, with the deadline for this income being Sunday. Before I did anything else, I sat down and visualized what would happen.

I perceived how good it would feel to have $1000 in such a short time, and I thought about the freedom this money would bring. I imagined how I would pay my bills with part of it and then spend the rest on a spa day.

I could see myself inserting my debit card into the ATM and paying a local business for their services, contributing to their livelihood. I sensed how good it would feel not to worry about the bills since I knew the money was in the bank. I imagined how great my nails would look after being freshly done at the spa.

After getting into this good emotional state, I got up and started working. I was now spiritually aligned and ready to get into action in my high vibrational state. I uploaded an ad on social media advertising a monthly virtual yoga class I was teaching on Zoom, and I added that registration was open. Within 3 hours, 12 people signed up which gave me $576. On Thursday and on Friday, I did the same thing and got into the spirit of having it done. On Friday, I got a cheque in the mail for an unexpected $500 with a reimbursement from the government.

I made a total of $1076. What I did was a manifestation of my goal. I visualized it, felt it completed, and then took the spiritually aligned action.

Let's break this down!

We'll begin with your goal. Please, write it again below. You can never put it down too many times!

Next, we'll get into the spirit of having it already done. Here is a visualization that you can do. For me, it works more effectively if I do it 1-3 times a day; in the morning, at lunchtime, and before I go to sleep.

- Play some soft music, maybe something that moves you in a really great way. Then, find a place where you can be quiet. It's optional if you keep the eyes open or closed. (Sometimes, I can visualize with my eyes open better than if I have them closed).
- Take a deep belly breath through your nose and let it slowly release through the mouth.
- As you exhale, feel your body soften.
- Allow your body to feel the support of the chair, bed, or floor below you.
- Continue to focus on your breath.
- Quiet your thoughts and bring your goal to the focus of your mind.

- See yourself with the goal fulfilled.
- What will you do once you achieve the goal? Who will be there around celebrating with you?
- What are you feeling? Are you feeling excitement, pride, or gratitude? Do you feel abundant? Do you feel love towards yourself? Are you accomplished and generous?
- Are you powerful and in control of your life?
- Add feelings to your goal.
- What are you doing with the money you'll make or the relationship you'll find?
- What does it mean to have your book written or to have a trip paid for? Lean into the feeling of it. Get specific and picture what you're wearing and how you're showing up.
- Paint the picture of the goal achieved clearly in your mind.
- Stay with it for a couple of moments. (I aim for at least 5-10 minutes).
- At the end of your visualization, say these words in your head or out loud, "and it is done" or "and so it is".
- Feeling 'as if' the goal is already achieved is getting you into a vibration of already having it done. It's called "becoming a vibrational match." We're no longer the caterpillar. We are now shifting to the energy of the butterfly!

Are you vibrating high? If not, you can use other methods to get into that higher vibration: music, dancing, going for a walk, hiking, loving up on your pet, grabbing your favorite cup of coffee, or going back to your list from our self-care chapter.

Shift the vibration, shift the vibration, shift the vibration.

Better? Good! Okay, now we step into the action piece. You may be thinking, "Kristy, where do I start?" I want to debunk some myths about "working hard", "I should be doing more" and "not doing enough."

My loves, here is what I've learned and I'm continuing to learn.

I used to have a full-time job and do between 10-30 hours of overtime. I also taught yoga classes trying to get ahead. What did I learn? Can anyone guess? I learned how to burn out fast. Sure, I felt accomplished, but really, where did it get me? I didn't have time for things I enjoyed; I built poor sleeping habits, and my health degraded. I'm sure you guessed what came next. More anxiety. Go, go, go, meant lots of thoughts like: "Did I remember to do that? Did I do it right? Oh god, I hope I make it on time. I was so busy I lost track of time. I can't be late."

"Well, that was a failure. I don't even feel present in this class. What a shit teacher I am."

So, that was fun! I no longer choose to believe that working all day every day will get me ahead. I trust and remember that beliefs are important and a couple of hours of solid, intentional, and spiritually aligned action are more effective.

Let's create a list of intentional actions you can do each day that will move you closer to your goal. Get specific, as always. There shouldn't be more than 5 items on the list.

These are solid intentional steps that you can take during your day.

1.

2.

3.

4.

5.

This list may change as you grow closer to your goal, and you may need to tweak it in order to make it support you more intentionally. Commit yourself to getting into the energy of the goal before taking these action steps. Dedicate yourself to doing at least 1 thing a day that will move you closer to your objective.

As I said, I believe that solid, intentional, and spiritually aligned action is more effective than long hours of unintentional, low-vibrational work. You can spend 30 minutes on intentional action, and it'll be more effective and efficient than an 8-hour workday. Everything is energy. We're energy. What we do has energy attached to it. We surround ourselves with other energetic beings, and we pass along and take on energy throughout the day. Ensure that the spirit you give to bring your objective closer is aligned with it.

Be intentional. Be aligned. Take action.

Let's move on to the next part of achieving our goal. The spiritually aligned action has been taken, and I'd like to take a few notes here. Please, don't get too attached to the outcome. What I want to say is that if your objective isn't reached by the deadline you've set, don't worry about it. Just keep holding the vision and be aware that it'll come.

That's easier said than done. I'm still working on this attitude of awareness myself. Please trust that even if it hasn't come yet, it doesn't mean it's not making its way to you.

Hold on to the deadline while feeling joyful expectation. It'll happen. Just keep aligning and taking action.

Now, we've reached the next point of our big, beautiful dream. After taking all the steps, I want you to let it go and release it.

Have I baffled you? Let's think this way: we can control our emotions, feelings, and decisions, but we can't be in charge of actions from the outside. It'll drive us crazy if we try to do it. Trust me, I've done it. For someone who has struggled with anxiety, control was something I held onto tightly. I wanted to decide about everything from the outside to make myself feel better. It took me a while, but finally I realized I didn't build my life based on the outside but on the inside.

We control our feelings, emotions, beliefs, and actions from the inside, and our outside should mirror them. What I'm trying to say is that if we try to control the goal from the outside by holding on tightly to the deadline and the outcome, we won't have any control over it.

What do you think is happening inside? We're feeling desperate and we wait longingly for something that hasn't happened yet. We're feeling the lack of our goal on the inside which as a result is mirrored on the outside.

The best advice I can give you is that at the end of your action steps, you should let the goal go to take its own form. Believe that what you've done today is enough, and you're closer to your objective. Surrendering allows the goal to show up in creative ways you've never even thought of.

Let's look again at my goal of $1000. If I were to say that I wanted $1000 solely from my yoga business before the end of the weekend, it wouldn't have happened in that time frame, and I would be okay with that. However, I took action and posted my ad on social media. I also let my goal go without thinking about failing, which didn't add any negative connotation to my aim. I just left it and felt in my body that it was already achieved. If I hadn't done that, I'd have limited myself.

I was open to getting $1000 in 5 days, and I didn't limit it by saying, "12 people signed up, and it isn't enough, I failed." I could have stressed about my objective and created a resistance that wouldn't have allowed the money to make its way to me, and maybe the $500 unexpected cheque wouldn't have appeared. It's creating the manifestation that helps us achieve our goals.

Letting go is important. You probably wonder what's the easiest way to do it. I want you to write down, maybe in a "bucket list" type of style, all the ways you can let go. It can be just telling yourself that your goal has been achieved every time that doubt seeps into your mind.

It could be distracting yourself with things and activities that bring you joy. Again, it's all about keeping yourself in a high vibrational state. Plan something with a friend or your partner.

Do a puzzle (when was the last time you did it?) or maybe built a Lego building. I used to think they were complicated and time-consuming when I was younger, but hey, they sure kept all my attention as I followed the directions to build them. That counts!

You may also try a new recipe, cook a meal that you always wanted to prepare, or pack your lunches for the following days. This way you won't constantly think about the goal, but you'll stay in the energy of the objective. It's a key to success! Do you remember that we attract that which matches our energy?

Why am I talking about goals in a book about mental illness? Objectives allowed me to redirect my focus and go through life with purpose. Having a goal not only did help to make my mindset shift to the life I wanted, but it also allowed me to LIVE the life I wanted. An aim gives us a sense of direction, an opportunity to grow and discover who the hell we are, and who we want to be. I wanted to live a luxurious, beautiful, and location-independent life, and I asked myself what I would need to do to achieve that. Well, I would be honing in on all I wished for and asking myself how I could serve people. I thought about all my experiences and passions that have changed my life and could be a light to guide others to change theirs.

I fully stepped into who I needed to be for myself and others. I set goals like having a $10,000 monthly income, which would allow me to make donations to foundations I believed in. I could buy gifts for my family and friends without any reason, take vacations, have all the bells and whistles added, and know I was worthy of it. I wanted to be a light for others, help them realize their potential, and make them see that there was so much more to live than one's diagnosis of mental illness. I wished to be an example of what was possible and show people how they could make their way out of the darkness and go back to the beautiful warmth of the light.

Set those big vibrant goals, my loves. You dreamed them up and you're meant to achieve them, otherwise you wouldn't have been gifted in seeing them in your mind. We were all born worthy of our dreams, our objectives, and purpose. All it takes is for you to be brave, to want to change and realize the big, scary, expansive dreams. I'm right there with you and I know you can do it. I think on some level you know that, too. The darkness was just a distraction from the ego to keep you from the love and light that you have to share.

Don't let it keep you small.

Go big, be bold.

Get excited about life.

Feel expansive.

We aren't thinking the caterpillar thoughts anymore.

You're ready to transform and bring out the butterfly. Get vibrantly colourful about those dreams!

I did it, and I'll never regret it, even for a second!

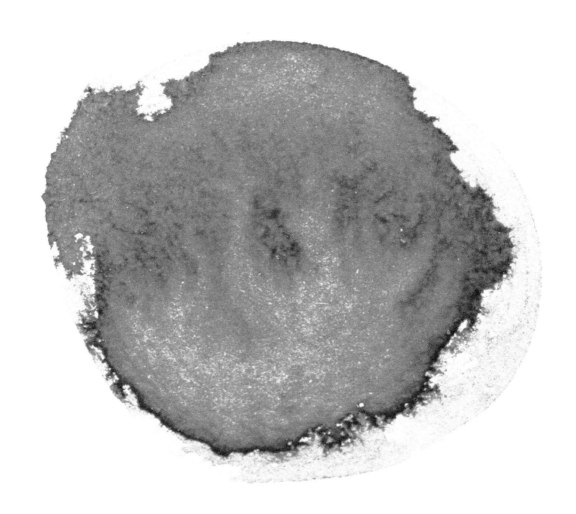

"You need to feel worthy from within."

Kylie

8

The Butterfly Show

Written with passion by Kylie

Picture this. You're trekking through the Sahara Desert. It's 40 degrees Celsius, and you've been walking for miles. The sun is beating down on you, and you have beads of sweat rolling down your forehead. You're carrying a heavy backpack with all your belongings, and you have one sip of water left in the water canister, which is supposed to get you through the day. You don't know where your next stop will be or how you will make it. I forgot to add that you also have a blister on your right heel, and no matter how you walk, you can't ease the pain for the life of you.

Do you think it sounds hard? Well, it isn't nearly as difficult as showing up for yourself. You might think I'm kidding, but I'm far from it. For some reason, people seem to really struggle with the concept of being there for themselves. You'll attend your best friend's daughter's dance recital. You'll go golfing with your boss, even though you don't golf. You'll watch your son walk across the stage for his preschool graduation. However, when it comes to being there for yourself, you're gone. Poof. It's like you were never even there to begin with.

I've recently signed up for Highland Dance. I know it sounds like a bizarre activity to randomly engage in. I did Highland Dance for years as a child and I participated in many competitions. When I was 15, I had to stop dancing because I developed an injury at a dance contest in New Hampshire that required surgery. After my medical procedure, I never went back to dancing because I was a teenager and I felt I was too cool to spin to bagpipes and a kilt.

However, as a 25-year-old woman married to her high school sweetheart, I decided I no longer needed to be cool, and I signed up for adult Highland Dance lessons. At the classes, my instructor, Brianna, informed me about an upcoming dance recital. Of course, I said I would participate! Even though it was supposed to be with a bunch of young children who were taking her other classes, I didn't care. I decided to turn this into a big event, and I invited family and friends to watch me prance around swords on stage with some kids.

During the weeks leading to the event, I missed a few dance classes because I felt low, anxious, tired, and overwhelmed with my life. I was in a generally low place, and I didn't want to go. So, I skipped some lessons. Those are the perks of being an adult. You can decide where you go and when you go. You choose how you show up and if you show up at all. I picked the second option.

As a result, I ended up bailing on the dance recital. I failed the dance teacher, the family that was coming to watch me, and my friends, who were excited to see this dance style in person for the first time. Most importantly, I let myself down because I couldn't show up for me, Kylie.

I used my mental health as an excuse — and while valid — sometimes it's a crutch that we rely on to get us out of things.

It may look impossible to push yourself forward when you're low. You may feel blind while you search for the end goal that's too far away to see. Why work for something now when the benefits aren't tangible or don't appear fast enough? How do we force ourselves to chase our dreams and accomplish tasks?

The simple answer is, you just do it. You just show up. There're some days when I can't even fathom the idea of emptying the dishwasher. For some reason, my husband is never around when it's time to do it, and if he's around, he never notices it is ready to be emptied. I view this as a tedious task, but I've done two things to make it easier, so I accomplish my goal of putting the dishes away.

The first thing I do is to tell myself that I'm just going to do a part of it. First, I'm going to put the cutlery away. That's it! It won't take long, and it isn't hard. If I feel like it later, I'll come back and do the top rack. Then, I can do the bottom rack. It might take me three different tries, but eventually the dishwasher will be empty.

What usually happens is that I end up putting away everything. Great! However, that's not the point. The idea is that if I can only complete what I set out to do, putting away the cutlery in my case, I'll still accomplish something and make progress. What I want to say is that we don't need to begin a task, get so involved in it, and just continue until the whole thing is done.

It's okay to do just a part that we can finish.

The second thing I do is to tell myself how much fun I have while putting the dishes away. I dread doing the task because I have this idea in my head that it sucks. But what if it doesn't? What if I put on my favorite song while I'm emptying the dishwasher? What if I convince myself how much I love it because then my house will feel clean, and I'll feel good?

Reframing the mindset has many benefits. Changing your thoughts from negativity and dread to positivity can have a profound impact on your ability to accomplish tasks, achieve goals, and reach your dreams.

Yes, I sound dramatic. Putting away dishes isn't me "achieving goals and reaching for dreams", but you can take this idea and this mindset and apply them to the areas of your life that signify something to you. At the end of the day, dishes don't mean a whole lot to me, but it's a small and easy way to practice showing up for myself so that I can do it when it really matters.

Another important point I'd like to mention is that we may not show up for ourselves because we feel insecure. We think we aren't worth it. I could sit here and tell you that in fact, you are worth it, but it doesn't matter what I think. You don't need external validation from me, some random woman who still microwaves most of her dinners and walks around the house chanting to her cats. What you need is internal validation.

You need to feel worthy from within. It's easier said than done, and learning to believe in it is a lifelong journey. You'll have days when you feel more confident. I believe that self-worth and self-love aren't something you ever accomplish fully, but it's a daily practice that you do to work towards your internal validation.

Here are some tips that we use to help us focus on feeling worthy from within:

- Every morning, I look at myself in the mirror and say three kind words before I start the day
- Throughout the day, any time I see myself in the mirror, I smile and say, 'you got this!'
- I practice kindness by talking to myself as if I'm one of my friends. I would never call my friend a failure or worthless. So, why am I okay to say those unhelpful comments to myself?
- I spend time focusing on self-care (see self-care chapter for more information)
- I focus on deep breathing throughout the day when I get overwhelmed or anxious and I feel I need to slow down. I remind myself

that I'm capable of handling any challenges that come my way.

- Try the 4-7-8 breathing method. Inhale for 4 counts. Hold for 7 counts. Exhale for 8 counts. Repeat. This exercise brings balance to your body and mind, helps you slow down, and it's effective in reducing stress and anxiety.
- Turn to gratitude. Repeat thank you 100 times when you get up. You can even start to be thankful for all you have. Thank your shower head for allowing you to bathe and thank your pillow for supporting your head while you sleep. Thank your coffee for filling the kitchen with a rich aroma and fueling you to jumpstart the day. Thank everything you encounter when you first get up and watch what attitude you'll have after.

Now, you may think that everything we're suggesting to you is way too hard.

You don't have enough time for that. You're right, it's hard! That's one of the reasons why it's so important for you. The more you do it, the more you practice showing up for yourself, and the easier it gets. Force the life you want until it becomes the life you have. To do this, you need to show up for yourself.

Another way you can show up for yourself is by showing up for others. It might surprise some people, but the coolest thing you can do is to show kindness. We live in a world that is full of disease, war, poverty, pandemic-related stressors, and daily tension. Why would we want to make life harder for ourselves and for others?

Supporting each other is critical for a thriving society. Caring for others is what helps small businesses survive, families raise children, and workers feel appreciated by their employer and colleagues. Without empathy, we'll live in a dog-eat-dog world, but with empathy we can build a world where everyone is able to fulfill their dreams. Our aspirations are within reach because anything feels possible.

Kristy's the creator of Defying Lee Fit, a business that focuses on yoga, wellness, and mindset. She's incredibly supportive of all women and truly believes there's room for everyone at the top. She's accomplished so many goals in her time and she's continuing to reach for the stars. My friend's a true inspiration and I can say this about her because she isn't writing this chapter. She's the kind of woman you want to be around. I'm telling you this because I've supported Kristy, and I want to use this as an example to demonstrate the importance of showing up for others and for yourself.

Kristy's sister, Chantel, is one of my best friends. Chantel and I met in the tenth grade, and we managed to keep our friendship strong for ten years despite her living in Ecuador for a bit and me living in France. I always knew Kristy and had her teach yoga at a Women's Day party I threw in 2019, but I'd never hung out with her on a personal level.

I decided to reach out to her because I'd been watching her on social media, and she was crushing it. She was a powerhouse woman who was putting herself in the world trying to help people make a difference in their lives. I could tell she wholeheartedly believed in everything she said and wanted to help people step into their full potential and reach their dreams. Kristy and I decided to do a couple of partnerships between Defying Lee Fit and Stella Jamieson Designs. They went well, and it was a mutual benefit. I felt inspired by Kristy to fulfill my aspirations.

I had always wanted to write a book, but I didn't know what it would entail, and the idea seemed daunting. It was something I wanted to achieve, but it didn't feel within reach.

However, I decided if I wished for it then I had to go for it, so I started writing.

While I was writing, I wanted to support Kristy in her upcoming workshop on Self Beliefs. She was excited and nervous to host the event, and I wanted to help her feel at ease because I knew she had so much to share with the world and she was going to do an incredible job.

Sometimes you just need support to help you recognize what you're capable of.

That's exactly what I noticed I needed, too.

The night of her workshop, I reached out to Kristy and asked her if she wanted to write a book with me. I sent her the chapters I'd already begun working on and held my breath while I waited for her rejection. It never came. I had supported Kristy on her ventures, and she had also encouraged me. This cooperation continued when she accepted my offer to work together on this book.

It turned out, just like me, Kristy had also always wanted to write a book! It felt like the stars were aligning for us, and some of our dreams were beginning to take shape.

Had we not been caring for each other by doing a few collaborations with our businesses, it probably wouldn't have led to us to work together on a book. It was the support we gave each other that helped us form a connection.

As you can see, networking is important, and it's been what inspired us to fulfill this goal of ours together. It's just the beginning! Kristy and I are just starting our lives, careers, this friendship, and business partnership. However, I know that it'll blossom into a magical journey because Kristy and I have both been there to support each other since day one.

With empathy, anything is possible.

It's because of the support that Kristy gave me with writing this book, that I felt like it was actually possible to do. I would start many books in the past, but I had never finished any of them. Kristy's assistance helped me realize I could do this. Watching Kristy show up for me, I showed up for myself, and incredible things began to happen.

It can feel daunting and terrifying. It can seem like a lot of hard work, but it's worth it. When you show up for yourself, you tell yourself you're worthy of success and accomplishment. You're deserving of reaching your goals and chasing your dreams. You're more likely to get where you want when you help others arrive at their destinations and when you show up for yourself. All you have to do is to show up.

"Regardless of what trauma you have faced, find a good counsellor you like. You are worth this investment."

Kylie

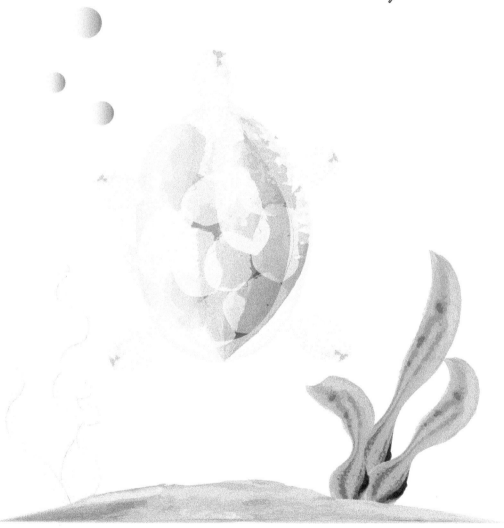

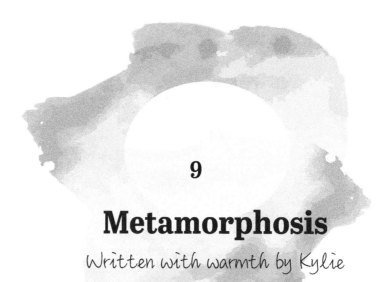

9

Metamorphosis

Written with warmth by Kylie

Trigger Warning: Sexual Assault, Self-Harm

It happened in July. My husband, Karl, and I, after being together for ten years, separated. We had been in a relationship since high school when we became high school sweethearts. I was 16, and I could hardly remember life without him. He was my best friend, and we had been through everything together. Now, he was gone.

The split was friendly and civil. We fought once, over who should keep our soft, plush towels. We both wanted them, but he was adamant that I should keep them even though I said he was the one who would take them. He taught me how to cut the grass before he left, because I'd never used a lawn mower before. He also talked to the neighbors to save me from awkward conversations about where he went and asked them to look out for me since I would be on my own.

Sometimes I wished we had fought. After all, it's easier to be mad than sad. Am I right? But I know how lucky we were to keep our friendship.

The funny thing about getting a divorce is that you can go down the rabbit hole of memories. There were many reasons we weren't meant to be together, but that didn't stop me from reminiscing on the good 'ol days. Our first group date of snowboarding and dining at East Side Mario's, walking home from school together, going to the drive-in together, and our family trip to Florida where we ate pizza for 2 weeks straight. We shared such fond memories but there would be no more to make.

One of the worst moments during the separation happened when I was working my second job. I took this position to keep my mind busy and receive some extra income. About six months prior, Karl and I had a joke where he called me a troll. He would put notes everywhere that said, "troll" on them. There was one I never found… until I was going through my bag at work and stumbled upon one of these "troll" notes.

That's the thing about a divorce, one minute you're fine and suddenly you're flooded with memories and pain. It can happen so unexpectedly.

I still haven't told my entire family about our separation. How do you explain that this man, who has done nothing wrong, but is no longer compatible with you as a life partner, won't be around anymore? I know I don't owe anybody an explanation, but that doesn't stop people from expecting one.

I let my anxiety get the best of me, and I worry. I worry about finances, the house I'm now responsible for, and our dog, Mocha, who we decided would be better off with Karl. My heart still aches for her. I hesitate if we've made the right decision (we have). I'm concerned about what people will say when they find out I'm dating again.

"Oh my gosh, it's so soon! Did she ever even love him? Did she cheat on him? Why did she move on so fast?"

Our marriage ended privately before it ended publicly. When we split up officially, we were ready to see other people. We lived together as friends, not lovers. There was no abuse or cheating. We were just companions. Simple as that. I know people would say I moved on quickly, so I had to actively tell myself that it wasn't important what they thought.

However, deep down, it did matter to me.

Months before Karl and I split, rumors circulated at my work about my sex life, and they destroyed my mental health. People thought I was sleeping with a married man while I was also married. That was far from the truth, but it wasn't the issue. What mattered was how this rumor circulated and escalated.

I allowed this false image of Kylie that people created to ruin me. When I downloaded a dating app and my colleagues started talking about my profile, I leaned on my friends to realize that people would talk. They'd think what they wanted, and I had no control over their thoughts. I could only be in charge of myself and my reactions.

The dating world was a place, unlike anything I'd ever experienced before. I felt like an alien walking on Earth for the first time. I was confident of my profile until a man pointed out I was wearing a wedding ring in all my pictures! My relationship had been in my life for so long that I didn't have any photos where I wasn't wearing either a promise ring, an engagement ring, or a wedding ring. Despite that, it was scrolling through men's pictures when I realized what my new life had become.

Almost every man had facial hair (I don't like facial hair). A lot of them showed their chests in pictures and some of them were oiled up... Many guys held fish in their photos, or showed images of them riding dirt bikes and driving boats. Most men would also put their height.

It wasn't their photos that was the interesting part but their personalities that they allowed to shine through. I had a man call me average looking and ask for a "pussy pic" in the same sentence. When I declined because I didn't send these type of photos, he then thought he would try his luck with an ass or tits snap. Blocked!

I became overwhelmed before I knew I was defeated. I wanted to enjoy my solo time, but a house can feel lonely, and the silence can be deafening. Swiping left or right can ease those feelings, but only temporarily.

I thought I was being safe, but I was far from it. A stranger asked me to drive 2 hours to the nearest city to meet him, bribing me with Ferrero Rocher, my favorite chocolate. It wasn't until I was all dolled up in the driver's seat of my car that I really listened to my friend screaming on the phone to get my ass back into the house. I work in the criminal justice system, for crying out loud, and I failed to see the danger in driving to some city to meet a random guy at a restaurant. I marched back into my quiet house and settled on the couch for the night, continuing to swipe from left to right. Potential disaster avoided! Thankfully, I had friends to rely on because I felt like I was drowning in the ocean, and I couldn't tell which way was up anymore.

Conversations can feel exhausting after a while. How often can you tell people about your hopes, dreams, goals, what you did today, or how you're doing, before it feels like a chore?

I began to look forward to the pick-up lines that arrived in my inbox because at least they were somewhat clever and put a temporary smile on my face. I had one match start a conversation by asking if I liked pineapple on my pizza. That was so much better than the conversations about how I was today blah blah blah. It was also a great way to get to know someone fast. You know, pineapple on pizza is a heated debate, and it can be a deal breaker.

It's always good to get that out of the way!

One day, somebody suggested a different dating app to me. There are so many different ones to choose from, but they're all relatively based on the same idea. You decide if the information somebody has entered (true or not) is worth your time. You fancy them or don't.

If you both like each other, you match, and then you can chat away about whatever your heart desires.

On this new dating app, I matched with a man named Tony. He was from the city, but he had a cottage near my place. Once we matched, he contacted me instantly. I didn't find this too odd because this had happened to me on the other site. It was Friday, and he was on the way to his cottage. He asked to meet me for coffee. That was it! Just a friendly conversation over a cup of coffee. I could do that, I thought.

When we arrived at the parking lot of the local coffee shop, he invited me into his truck. The first thing I noticed about his vehicle was that he had a sticker supporting breast cancer research. He couldn't be that bad a guy, right? The first thing I said to him when I entered his truck was that I loved how he was a supporter, and he talked to me about his sister who had breast cancer.

We chatted for a bit, getting to know each other better. I was interested in learning about him. I could feel his gaze on me, but it didn't make me uncomfortable. It just felt... noticeable. Perhaps this is what they call a red flag, I wasn't sure. I was so unfamiliar with the dating world that everything felt uncomfortable. How could I trust my gut when I didn't know what his behavior meant?

You know the part in horror movies when the characters are walking toward the bad guy, and you're screaming: "NO! NO! NO! DON'T GO!"? Well, this was that part for me. In the seat of his truck, he looked at me like I was an object, a piece of meat, and I was his. As a feminist, I thought I had a pretty good idea of how sex-driven men would behave. Boy, was I wrong! Watching him devour me with his eyes had the hairs on the back of my neck standing.

"No" is a word a 3-year-old can understand, but a grown man can't. Without going into graphic details, because my mind can't process that yet, he raped me. When he finished, I drove to the drugstore and bought condoms. It was too late for that, but I felt like I had to do something. The cashier asked me if I wanted a bag. I smiled and declined. How normal I was after such a traumatic event, I thought! I didn't allow myself to think about what had just happened.

Then, I drove to the hospital.

I grabbed a parking ticket and entered the Emergency Department. A triage nurse took me into their room and asked what brought me in.

"I was raped.", my voice cracked. She asked me to repeat what I had just said, so I squeezed my eyes shut tight and echoed my words quietly. When I opened my eyes, tears were streaming down my cheeks. The nurse was looking at me with love and pain in her eyes. We held each other's gaze for a few moments, and it felt like it was just the two of us in the room, acknowledging how shitty it was to be a woman sometimes.

Then, the hustle bustle began.

The nurses brought me cookies, ginger ale, and juice. They held me, hugged me, and cried with me. They also stayed around while I called a friend. They arranged for me to go to the nearest Sexual Assault Centre located at a hospital an hour away from the Emergency Department. They nested me in a cocoon of their love, sheltering me, keeping me safe, and expressing tender compassion. When I forgot where I had put my parking pass in all the chaos going on in my mind, they helped me leave the premises without it.

The nurse I met at the Sexual Assault Centre was incredible. She, too, had compassion and kindness in her voice while she walked me through the process.

I don't wish this experience upon anyone, but, based on my case, remember that the healthcare system makes sure you're looked after if you find yourself in this situation. Depending on what you need, they can provide you with medication to prevent pregnancy and sexually transmitted infections. They also have an abundance of resources to help you with support and counselling after the event.

A lot of women fear the legal system in cases like this for many reasons. Nobody wants to explain their story repeatedly, or have holes poked in it. Nobody wants to hear they are lying, they shouldn't have put themselves in that situation, or that they asked for it. These are the reasons why I decided to make a statement to the police, but not proceed with a report .

I value my mental health over anything else, and I couldn't put myself in a situation where my actions and decisions were questioned. I know that I made a mistake going out with that guy, but I didn't ask for this.

The first recommendation I have for anyone going through a situation like this, is to get counseling. Regardless of what trauma you have faced, find a good therapist. You're worth this investment! Sometimes you just need to talk things out and having someone help to guide your thoughts and unravel them, can show you how to process them and to better rationalize.

I needed to learn how to manage my emotions when I wasn't with my therapist. Counseling might last an hour each week, but then we need to face the rest of the hours. I found a beautiful notebook, and I used it to write about my thoughts each day. If I felt anxious about my job, I wrote it down. If I felt responsible for putting myself in a bad situation, I wrote it down. If I felt lonely, I wrote it down. Building this habit for my feelings helped me get them out of my head and allowed me to see the bigger picture.

It also helped me to explore different emotions. Instead of saying "I'm mad right now", I could find what was behind that sensation. Was I betrayed? Was I disrespected?

Was I provoked? Was I withdrawn? What feelings were really behind the core emotion of my anger? Once I was aware of that, I could better understand what had caused my reaction, and then I could target it. (See the chart at the end of this chapter to help you with your feelings.)

It's important to develop healthy coping techniques. For years, I leaned on self-harm as a coping technique, and I still find myself engaging in this unhealthy method when I feel out of control. In your case it may be overeating, starving, drugs, alcohol, or even isolating. Developing a list of healthy coping techniques that work well for you is beneficial when you want to rely on your old ways. When you're in the heat of the moment, and you want to engage in unhealthy coping mechanisms, you can look at your list and try some of the positive coping techniques that have helped you in the past.

Be mindful of your coping techniques. While they might work sometimes, it's not the best idea to use the same coping method all the time. For example, talking to a friend may be something that works for you; however, you don't want every conversation you have with them to focus on your current struggles. Therefore, finding various coping techniques will be beneficial for you and those around you.

Here are some ideas that could be useful for you:

- Painting
- Walking/hiking
- Manicure or pedicure
- Exercise (biking, lifting weights, yoga, swimming)
- Meditation
- Colouring
- Deep breathing
- Writing a journal
- Bubble bath

- Challenging irrational thoughts
- Listening to a positive song or podcast

Find a balance between "me time" and socializing. It's important to get out and see friends, but it's just as crucial to take time for yourself to heal, rest, do nothing, or just process. Don't be ashamed if you need time to do this, just embrace it and lean into it, but don't forget about your friends, either. Positive relationships can help immensely with supporting you with what you need at the present moment, and getting you out of any ruts you may find yourself in.

Writing Activity

Write down a story that you've been bottling up. Let it all out! (Use the next page or a favorite journal to jot down your thoughts to the following questions)

What happened?

How did you feel? Really explore these emotions with the Feelings Chart on the

following pages.

Why have you kept this a secret?

What did you learn?

What coping strategies have helped you through?

My Story:

_____
_____
_____
_____
_____
_____
_____
_____
_____
_____
_____
_____
_____
_____
_____
_____
_____
_____
_____
_____
_____
_____

The Feelings Chart (Part I)

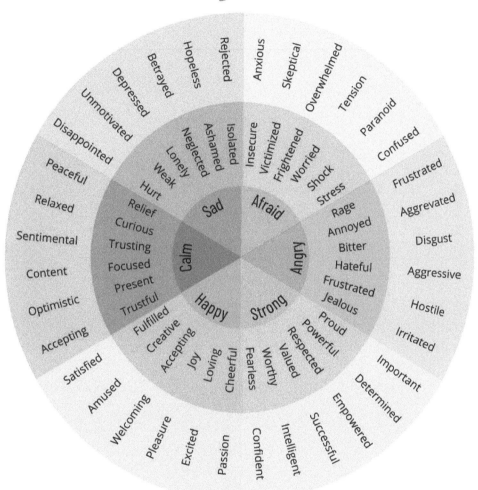

To quickly evaluate your story (previous activity), and help you better identify your emotional range during any given day/event/experience, refer to our Feelings Charts (Part I and Part II)

The Feelings Chart (Part II)

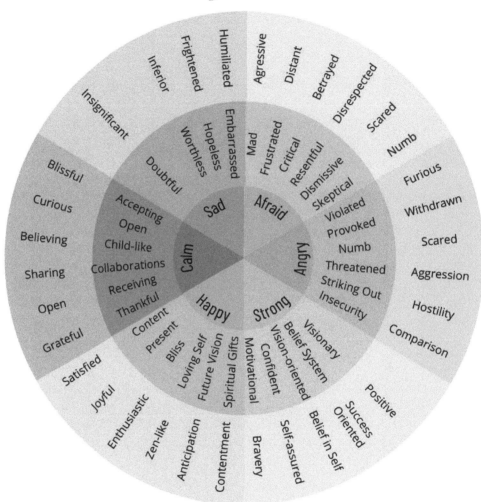

Sexual Assault Resources Ontario

Assaulted Women's Helpline

1-866-863-0511

Victim Support Line

1-888-579-2888

Fem'aide

1-877-336-2433

Talk4Healing

1-855-554-4325

"Your life can be as full as you desire it,

you just have to have faith enough to go for it."

Kristy

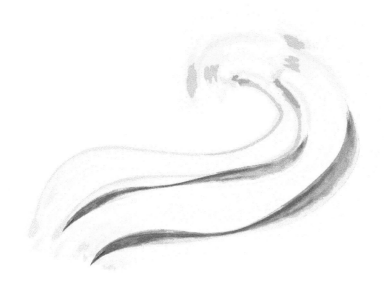

10

The Butterfly Comes After the Cocoon

Written with faith by Kristy

Faith has been a more recent endeavor for me. When someone talked about faith in the past, I was immediately turned off and wanted nothing to do with any part of this conversation. When listening to a talk about religion, my mind would automatically goes to super pious people who believed in a man with a beard. Someone that I didn't give credence to. Many years passed before I could realize that I was a part of a greater consciousness and we were all connected to the oneness of spirit and all things.

My first experience with a greater consciousness came to me when I was at my breaking point. I was experiencing a moment of such darkness that I couldn't bear it any longer.

My life wasn't improving, and I felt it would never get better. I made a decision to end it all.

I just didn't want to live anymore. I was in my last year of university, and the force of what was coming was sitting like bricks on my chest, crushing and holding me paralyzed in fear. With only a couple of months before my final examinations, I couldn't stand the pressure, and felt an impending failure.

I decided to walk out of my apartment, get on a public bus, and go to the pharmacy.

The snow had just dusted the ground. It was cold, and the wind cut through my winter jacket.

I walked, passing the brick buildings that housed families and students just like me. I trudged down the street, turned left and then turned right to go to the bus stop. I rode the bus into town and then took another one to Walmart. I got off there and went straight to the pharmacy section.

I was acting on autopilot. My mind was looking for something to make all the feelings go away. I didn't want to perceive anymore. I just wanted to numb out or go to sleep. Permanently…

I was trying not to tremble and to breathe normally. My nose was running, and I was struggling to focus on the pill bottles through my blurred vision as I held back tears. It would be better this way, I told myself. I wanted no more suffering. I could just be free from the anxiety at last. I grabbed a smorgasbord of bottles, not knowing exactly what might work. I felt eyes staring at me as if people knew what I was there for, so I hurried and moved away from the aisle.

At this point, I was shaking, and my whole body was vibrating. I was scared. I kept repeating under my breath that it would all be put to rest soon. I was afraid of myself, and I just wanted to quiet the noise. To be finally at peace. I walked down the store aisle heading toward the cashier's checkout counter.

I had a moment of clarity, and a little voice in my head came out of nowhere. It told me to **"STOP"** so I halted my prompt stride. I was breathing heavily, unsure of the sudden ringing I heard. I felt an urge, as if I was being called to the book section. It was weird, right? Still gripping all the bottles in my hands, I turned and followed the calling. I walked up to the display, grazing my eyes over the selection. I saw a book. It was the book I'd been looking for as a recommendation from my counselor.

Something inside told me to buy this book. I left all the bottles on the display, picked up this tiny novel, and went to pay for it. I felt so much shame about what I'd intended to do.

The tears began to flow uncontrollably, but the little voice made itself known again and said: "forgive yourself and read this book." I took a deep breath and felt incredible love toward myself. I experienced this overwhelming amount of tenderness and support as I stood in the middle of the book section. People were watching me with concern, but all I cared about was the voice in my head telling me: "Love yourself. Think bigger than this. You are extraordinary, and you just need to get past this moment."

The book was **The Four Agreements by Don Miguel Ruiz**. I left the store, my tiny book locked in my grip, and went home, and read the entire book that afternoon. I used to say that this little publication saved my life, but now I know it was my inner consciousness. If I listened to this part of me that wanted a better life, then I could get through this. And I could get through almost anything!

It's how it all started for me, and my faith began to grow. I'd get quiet and listen to that inner voice as it guided me. I knew that if I turned away from fear (ego) and tuned into loving voices, I would see what my world could look like. Faith to me was this absolute knowledge that everything was going to work out okay, and all I wanted in this life would come to fruition if I believed it was possible. It took quite a bit of will power to stay focused on the loving side of my thoughts and desires and not to return to my instinctual and habitual thinking based on fear and lack. However, the more I practiced faith, the more things started to show up, presenting me with opportunities to create things I always wanted to do.

I graduated from university with minimal stress and made the Dean's Honours list.

I trusted I would eventually find my calling, so I let go of the shame of my mistakes and the jobs I took while I was being guided to my purpose. I also stopped the judgment I placed on myself and those around me.

After I trained myself to lean more into faith, more life came into my life. I could experience it, better yet, I could enjoy it. When you feel guided and believe that your journey is unfolding **FOR** you, what is there to worry about? Mind you, all this didn't happen overnight. Sometimes I'd lean into ego thoughts and give credence to the worrying images that popped in my mind. Then, I had to shift back into my faith. It's like a muscle; we need to practice using it and give it the right form and alignment so that it could become stronger. I had to refuse dark thoughts come through and tell me that life wasn't good or it wasn't for me. Instead, I needed to push through and convince myself that it would get better, and if I focused on the good, then it would come.

I believed I was meant for more. My life was full, and I could have adventures and go after the things I wanted. As a result, more positive events occurred.

Later, I took a yoga teacher training. It scared me to death, but I had faith I could manage it, and allowed myself to embrace the experience. It led me deeper into my faith.

I wanted to bring this practice to more people, so I figured it all out by myself. I learned how to film, edit, and create an online studio for persons from all over the world to access my classes. I created programs to share how I redefined my anxiety and to show others how to do the same and create a life beyond their wildest dreams.

All this came about because I had faith. I believed that if I had the idea; I was meant to fulfill it, and I would be guided to bring it from my imagination to its physical form. I could have let those fearful and doubtful thoughts impede my mind and become paralyzed, but instead I chose to persevere and bring my dreams to life.

For example, think about how this book came about. I was talking to a relative on a Friday while I was driving home, and I said: "I am feeling called to write a book about my story, but I don't know if it's the right time because I have so much going on." I was about to get all flustered, but then I thought, "Well, I'll leave it up to the universe. If I'm meant to write a book now, I'll be open to a sign to tell me so." I just stopped giving it attention. I taught yoga all weekend, spent time with family, and didn't give it another thought. On Monday, Kylie messaged me, asking if I'd ever considered writing a self-development book.

Well, if that isn't a sign from the universe, I don't know what is!

Of course, I excitedly said yes! So, here we are, meeting with our publisher, finding an illustrator, and setting the book in motion. If I didn't trust that the book would happen and let go of the timeline, I would probably still be hemming and hawing about it. Faith is seeing your goal crystal clear and trusting that it'll show up as you pictured it or even better than you imagined. I truly believe everything happens for a reason, my path is constantly guided, and I am co-creating with a greater force.

Faith can look any way you want it to look. I used to get hung up on this word and concept of God, but when I think of my spirituality, I resonate with the language of the Universe. Whatever it is; Spirit, God, Higher Self, Universe, The Divine, we're all tapping into that force and constantly co-creating with it, whether for the good or the bad. I feel comforted knowing that when I need a sign, I'll see it.

A couple of weeks ago, I woke up with anxiety about my business and money. I had to stop that thought in its tracks and take a breath. Then, I silently said, "Universe, please give me my sign to let me know I'm on the right path." I let it go, and then I went to teach a dock yoga class. After finishing my session, I was chit-chatting with the group when I saw an "fox" written on a woman's shirt. (You need to know that I always ask to see a fox as my sign.)

It stopped my train of thoughts, and I asked her, "Excuse me, does your sweater say fox?"

She replied, "Yes, it's White Fox Soccer." I told her my story about asking to see that sign, and she said, "I had a different shirt on when I left the cottage, but then I turned around and went back inside to change." She told me she didn't know why but felt pulled to do it.

My heart was so full, the universe answered in just a few short hours. If you want to be guided, ask for a sign, pick something that resonates with you. It could be an animal, a coloured feather, or something else. Just ask to see it within 24 to 48 hours. You can be lead, if you're ready for it. Open yourself up to the universe (or the language of the source you choose) and see literal magic unfold before you.

Now, try this exercise.

Choose your sign and proclaim powerfully to the universe that you'd like to see it within 48 hours regarding your question. To solidify it, I recommend you write it down. A sticky note, or in a notepad works fine.

Another way to connect to the source is to get into a meditative state. Choose an activity, whether sitting, listening to soothing music, going for a silent car ride, or taking an unplugged walk. The action should quiet your mind, so you can make room for that inner voice and hear it speak wisdom to and through you. If an idea comes to you, no matter how big or small, it's because you're capable of doing it. If you see yourself driving that sports car, you can achieve to own it. If you see yourself horseback riding, you have the skill to do it. If you see yourself running a business, you're guided to figure it out and take steps to be your own boss. Don't ignore it because you feel scared, but take action, trusting that it'll all work out in the way it's meant to be. We're in constant co-creation of our lives, my friends, so open yourself up to receive and then act on the guidance. Your life can be as full as you desire, you just need to have enough faith to go for it.

Here are some affirmations that you can use, anytime your faith waivers.

~ I AM GUIDED IN EACH MOMENT ~

~ THE UNIVERSE HAS MY BACK ~

~ I CHOOSE _____ OR SOMETHING BETTER ~

~ I HAVE FAITH THAT IT WILL WORK OUT FOR THE HIGHEST GOOD FOR ALL ~

~ I WAS GIVEN THIS IDEA, AND I TRUST THAT IT WAS MEANT FOR ME ~

~ I CHOOSE TO LEAN INTO FAITH AND LOVE ~

~ IF I KEEP MY GOAL IN THE FOREFRONT OF MY IMAGINATION, THAN I TRUST IT WILL COME INTO FRUITION THROUGH MY CO CREATION WITH THE UNIVERSE. ~

The way affirmations work is to remind us of them and make us feel them. It won't be effective if you say an affirmation on autopilot without registering what it means for you. Allow yourself to feel the connotation of that affirmation. For instance, think how it makes you feel to know this: "If I keep my goal in the forefront of my imagination, then I trust it'll come to fruition through my co-creation with the universe." What do these words represent for you?

For me, it means: "You're a wizard, Harry". Seriously, if you can create a scene in your mind and then go out to the world acting in faith that it'll come true, that's magic. Real-life magic! Generate the feeling and allow these affirmations to remind you that you're amazing, and the universe is creating your dream life. It'll all come together!

Things to be Grateful for

Animals with four legs • Chocolate • Sunshine • Rainbows • The fizz in pop • Drums • Candles • Butterflies • Rainstorms • Snowflakes • Gnomes • Science • High heels • Workout classes • Winter tires • Drive-thru with no line-up • Mail from an old friend • Surprises • Rollercoasters • The ocean • Airplanes • Social service workers • Job interviews • Yoga • Halloween • Mugs with funny sayings • Crystals • Christmas lights • Meditation • Dogs dressed in clothes • Salt lamps • Windshield wipers • Laughing children • Hot tubs • Bath bombs • Purple pens • Comfy pants • Sunscreen • Sporks • Freshly squeezed lemonade • Crisp fall air •Thanksgiving turkey • Cardigans • The smell of grass • Gooey chocolate chip cookies • Naps • Pretty journals • Concerts • Iced coffee • Traffic lights • Your favorite song • Quotes by wise people • Soft blankets • Roller skates • Health • Toothpaste • Tacos • Bumblebees • Art • Campfires • Stargazing • Movie theatres • Bakeries • Smoothies • Smiles from strangers • Icing • Laughter • Sprinklers • Your home • Glasses • Comedians • Sunsets • Chapstick • Eyeliner • Confetti • Stress balls • Dolphins • Cue cards • Friends • Cuddling • Broadway • Poetry • Polymer clay earrings • Positive people • Fire hydrants • Opportunities • Sandy beaches • Fruit • Garbage collectors • Video calls • Smores • Carnivals • Museums • Hammocks • Comfy beds • A favorite t-shirt • Horror movies •

What are you grateful for?

Mini-Workbook

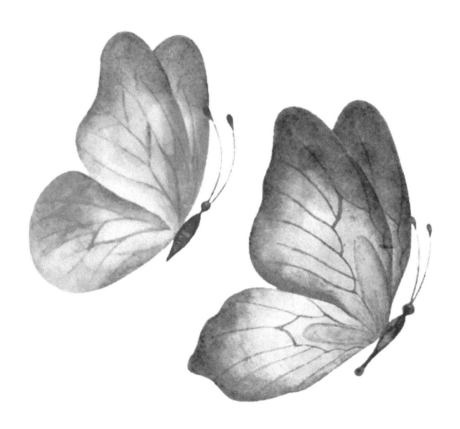

Affirmations

Anything I desire can and will be mine

I radiate power

I am prosperity

I am safe; I am secure; I am loved; I am enough, and even though _____ is happening right now, I deeply and completely love and accept myself

I get to decide how my day goes

I choose to be a light today for myself and others

Everything happens in divine timing; I am guided to all that is FOR me

I have the power within me to create my reality. I am the

cause to my effect

I feel good at this moment

I am in constant abundance and overflow. I have more than enough

Nothing outside of me can affect me without my permission

I choose to find miracles every single day.my effect

I feel good at this moment

Self-Love

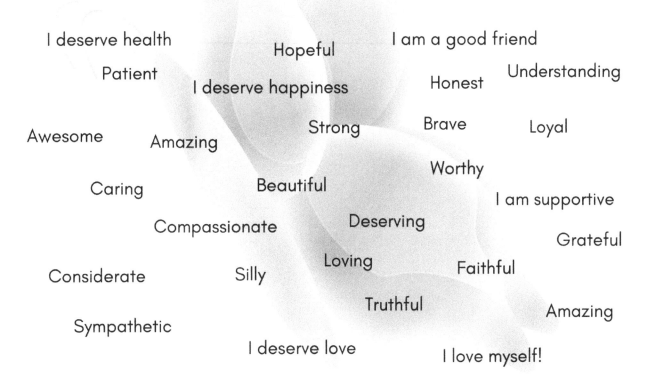

I deserve health

Hopeful

I am a good friend

Patient

Understanding

I deserve happiness

Honest

Strong

Brave

Loyal

Awesome

Amazing

Worthy

Caring

Beautiful

I am supportive

Compassionate

Deserving

Grateful

Loving

Considerate

Silly

Faithful

Truthful

Amazing

Sympathetic

I deserve love

I love myself!

Write a love letter to yourself about all your amazing traits and read it out loud when you're low.

ou may feel silly at first, but it's helpful to encourage you to acknowledge your strengths. Feel free to use some of our suggested, power-words.

Relaxation Exercises

Light stretching

Shoulder rolls

Move your head in circles

Move wrists and ankles in circles

Massage temples

Run wrists under cold water

Listen to relaxing music

Breathwork

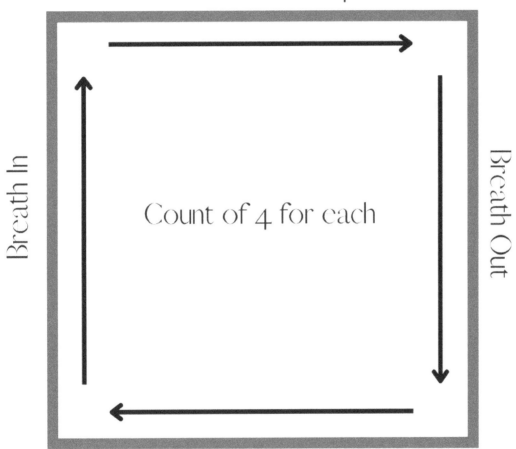

Hold at the top

Breath In

Count of 4 for each

Breath Out

Hold at the bottom

Color Me

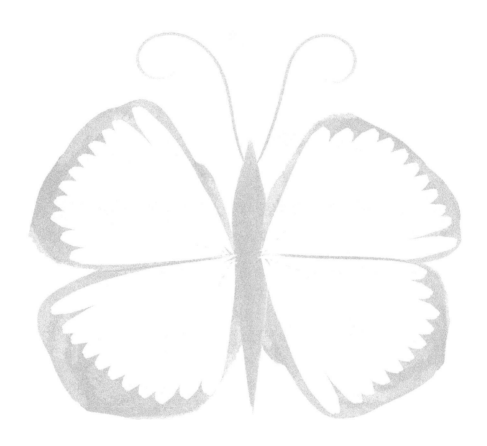

Write. It doesn't have to make sense. It doesn't need to be in complete sentences. Writing can help you understand your deepest thoughts and allow you to let go of your troubles.

Stress Response Exercise

What are some sources of your stress?

(Example: fighting with your parents)

What are some areas in your life that make you happy?

(Example: a yummy meal)

What are some healthy coping techniques that work well for you?

(Example: exercise)

What are some protective factors in your life that protect you from stress?

(Example: health, support system)

Relaxation Exercises

Light stretching

Shoulder rolls

Move your head in circles

Move wrists and ankles in circles

Massage temples

Run wrists under cold water

Listen to relaxing music

Deep breathing

"When it feels too hard to go on, be kind to yourself."

Kylie

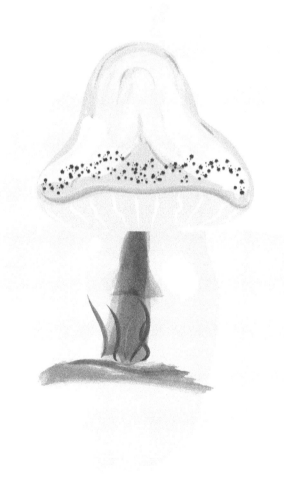

Conclusion

Acaterpillar goes through a metamorphosis to become a butterfly. to go through that process, it transforms itself into a chrysalis. This task takes approximately 14 to 18 days.

For humans, this is a remarkable transformation that can take much longer. However, like a caterpillar, we emerge as a butterfly once we have transformed.

The work to become a butterfly isn't an easy quest. There will be blood, sweat, and tears, and work will never truly stop. It takes perseverance, drive, motivation, and determination to live every day as the butterfly you are meant to be.

Sometimes it will feel harder than usual. There will be days when you'll feel like you've just begun the process, even though you've been doing it for ages. There will be days when the inner work seems daunting, and it's easier to stay a caterpillar. However, there will also be days when you'll relish the beautiful person you've become and be grateful for the effort you've been putting in.

When it feels too hard to go on, be kind to yourself. Go through the tips we've suggested in this book and tackle one thing at a time. Start by covering your basics. Have you showered? Have you eaten? Have you slept enough? Have you had enough water? Once you cover the essentials, you can move on to the inner work of believing in yourself, trusting the process, finding, and living within your purpose, and becoming the butterfly you are meant to be.

What if it all feels too hard? Flip back to the chapter on **Loving It Up And Feeling Good**. Self-care is extremely important because the work you're doing isn't easy. It isn't simply to transform and challenge yourself and your ideals. Pause and be proud of yourself.

Treat yourself with kindness.

You read about the challenges we'd gone through to work on becoming the best versions of ourselves. It's an everyday process. If you take some of our tips and tricks that work well for you, you can become a beautiful, tranquil, magical, majestic, unique, and individual butterfly, too.

Now go on, butterfly, and fly.

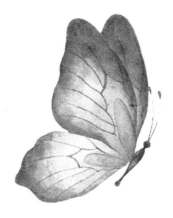

A Special Thank you to...

with love from Kylie

MY PARENTS AND SIBLINGS for supporting all my whacky ideas... or at least understanding there's no point in talking me out of it, because I'm going to do it anyway.

Christine Bell, Rebecca Fast, and Jasmine Swadia for being true friends, always showing up to support me, and hyping me up when I'm low.

Karl Koner for understanding that, like Miley Cyrus, I can't be tamed, and for watching with admiration as I strive to reach my dreams. I appreciate your endless support and friendship.

Michelle Lucas, my work mom, thank you for always making time, always listening without judgement, always supporting, and always having my back.

You're a true inspiration, and I admire you so much.

Kristy, for being so easy to write with and for making this journey such an enjoyable process. There's nobody else I'd rather write a freaking book with than you, my dear!

And, to one special person who should not be named... you know who you are.

Finally, to me... for believing in myself and my dreams, and doing everything I can to accomplish my goals.

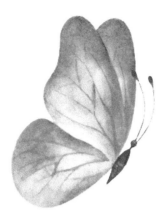

A Special Thank you to...

with love from Kristy

MY MOM, DEBBIE, for always being there for me as a powerhouse badass woman, and a role model for me, my brother and sister.

My Dad, Wayne, for encouraging me to follow my dreams, keep going, and showing me what is possible when I believe in myself.

My Sister, Chantel for always listening to my crazy ideas and going along for the ride. For being my confidant and best friend.

My Brother, Braedon, for always supporting everything I do, no matter how wild or out there it may seem. So grateful you are my brother, I hope this book inspires you.

My partner in love, Trish, for being my person to dream big with, my co-creator in this life, and one of my biggest cheerleaders.

Kylie, for being an answer to my prayer from the Universe to get our story out there. You inspire me and make me so proud of our partnership.

My Aunt Jackie, for supporting my big dreams and always connecting, building, and being there when I need it.

Connect with Us

Connect with us, scan the QR-Code to stay up-to-date with us, and our activities through Instagram, and on-line.

LOVE our book? Please consider leaving us a review on Amazon!

We are so grateful for your support,

Kristy and Kylie!

We have just begun...

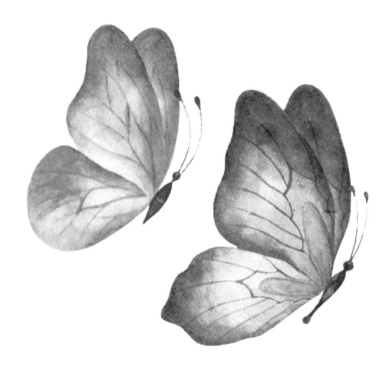

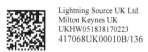

Lightning Source UK Ltd.
Milton Keynes UK
UKHW051838170223
417068UK00010B/136